Meta-Health

Sonali Vyas • Sunil Gupta • Abhishek Tyagi

Meta-Health

Understanding Metaverse for Healthcare

Springer

Sonali Vyas
School of Computer Science
University of Petroleum & Energy Studies (UPES)
Dehradun, Uttarakhand, India

Sunil Gupta
School of Computer Science
University of Petroleum & Energy Studies (UPES)
Dehradun, Uttarakhand, India

Abhishek Tyagi
Senior Formulation Scientist, Research and Development, King's Flair International (Holdings) Limited
Melbourne, VIC, Australia

ISBN 978-981-96-5843-5 ISBN 978-981-96-5844-2 (eBook)
https://doi.org/10.1007/978-981-96-5844-2

This Springer imprint is published by the registered company Springer Nature Singapore Pte Ltd.
The registered company address is: 152 Beach Road, #21-01/04 Gateway East, Singapore 189721, Singapore

Preface

The healthcare industry has been undergoing a transformative shift with the rapid advancements in digital technologies. From telemedicine and artificial intelligence to blockchain and the Internet of Medical Things (IoMT), digital health innovations have significantly improved patient care, diagnostics, and treatment. However, the emergence of the metaverse marks the beginning of a new era that integrates immersive virtual experiences with healthcare, creating what we now term as Meta-Health.

Meta-Health represents the convergence of metaverse technologies—such as augmented reality (AR), virtual reality (VR), extended reality (XR), mixed reality (MR), and blockchain—with healthcare services and applications. This paradigm shift is poised to revolutionize patient engagement, clinical training, remote diagnostics, and even therapeutic interventions. By harnessing immersive and decentralized digital ecosystems, healthcare can become more accessible, interactive, and personalized than ever before.

This book, *Meta-Health: Understanding Metaverse for Healthcare*, aims to provide a comprehensive exploration of the role of the metaverse in shaping the future of healthcare. The chapters in this book systematically cover various aspects of Meta-Health, offering insights into its technological foundations, applications, and future potential.

Chapter 1: Metaverse and its Applications lays the groundwork by discussing the evolution of the metaverse and its impact across industries, particularly in healthcare.

Chapter 2: Revolution of Healthcare Industry highlights key technological breakthroughs that have led to the digital transformation of healthcare.

Chapter 3: Meta-Health and Its Understanding delves into the definition, scope, and practical implications of Meta-Health in medical and healthcare practices.

Chapter 4: Technologies Enabling Meta-Health examines the cutting-edge technologies driving Meta-Health, such as AI, blockchain, IoMT, and cloud computing.

Chapter 5: Meta-Health Digital Therapeutic Applications explores the use of digital therapeutics in virtual healthcare environments, offering new treatment modalities for chronic diseases and mental health.

Chapter 6: Role of AR/VR/XR/MR in Meta-Health investigates how immersive technologies enhance medical training, patient engagement, and virtual consultations.

Chapter 7: Meta-Health Data Privacy and Security addresses the challenges and solutions related to securing sensitive patient data in the digital realm.

Chapter 8: Mimicking Healthcare in Meta-Health explores how real-world healthcare environments can be replicated within the metaverse for simulations, medical training, and telemedicine.

Chapter 9: New Business Models for Meta-Health provides insights into emerging revenue streams and economic structures within Meta-Health ecosystems.

Chapter 10: Future of Meta-Health presents potential advancements, ethical considerations, and regulatory frameworks that will shape Meta-Health in the coming years.

This book is designed for healthcare professionals, technologists, researchers, policymakers, and entrepreneurs seeking to understand and leverage the opportunities presented by Meta-Health. By bridging the gap between healthcare and the metaverse, we envision a future where medical services transcend physical limitations, fostering better patient outcomes, enhanced clinical collaboration, and democratized access to healthcare solutions.

This book serves as a valuable resource in understanding the profound impact of the metaverse on the future of healthcare. May it inspire innovation, drive discussions, and contribute to shaping a more connected and immersive healthcare ecosystem.

Dehradun, Uttarakhand, India — Sonali Vyas
Dehradun, Uttarakhand, India — Sunil Gupta
Melbourne, VIC, Australia — Abhishek Tyagi

Contents

About the Authors

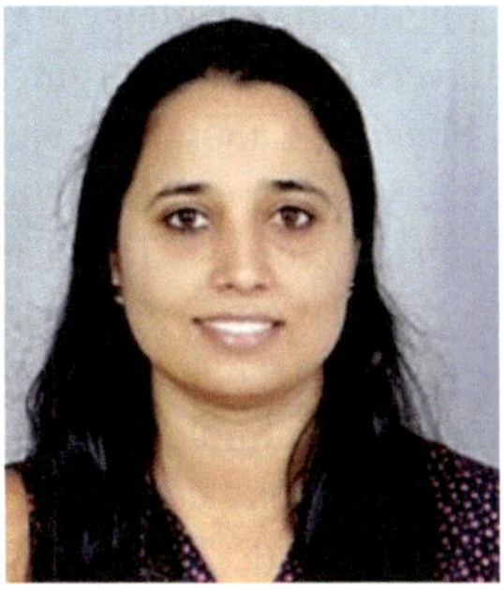

Sonali Vyas, Ph.D. is an accomplished academician and researcher with over 14 years of experience in the field of Computer Science. Currently serving as an Associate Professor in the School of Computer Science at the University of Petroleum and Energy Studies, Uttarakhand, Dr. Vyas has made significant contributions to Healthcare Informatics, Data Science, Database Virtualization, Data Mining, and Data Analytics. She is Senior Member-IEEE, Member ACM-India, Life Member-CSI, IFERP, IAENG, ISOC, SCRS, and IJERT.

She has an extensive publication record, with over 120 research papers, articles, and book chapters to her name in esteemed journals, conference proceedings, and books. Dr. Vyas is the author of the book *Smart Health Systems* published by Springer and has edited several influential works, including *Computational Intelligence in Urban Infrastructure* (CRC Press), *Handbook on Augmenting Telehealth Services: Using Artificial Intelligence* (CRC Press), *Blockchain Technology: Exploring Opportunities, Challenges, and Applications* (CRC Press), *Pervasive Computing: A Networking Perspective and Future Directions* (Springer Nature), and *Smart Farming Technologies for Sustainable Agricultural Development* (IGI Global).

Dr. Vyas has demonstrated innovation through the authorship of four patents focused on smart and sustainable systems. She has also been an influential voice in her field, delivering talks at both national and international conferences and serving as a resource person for AICTE-ISTE Faculty Refresher Courses on topics such as Embedded Systems, IoT, and Pervasive Computing.

Her commitment to academic excellence is further reflected in her membership on various editorial and review boards of respected national and international journals. She has actively contributed to the organization of numerous conferences, serving on organizing committees, national advisory boards, and technical program committees, and has chaired sessions at distinguished conferences worldwide.

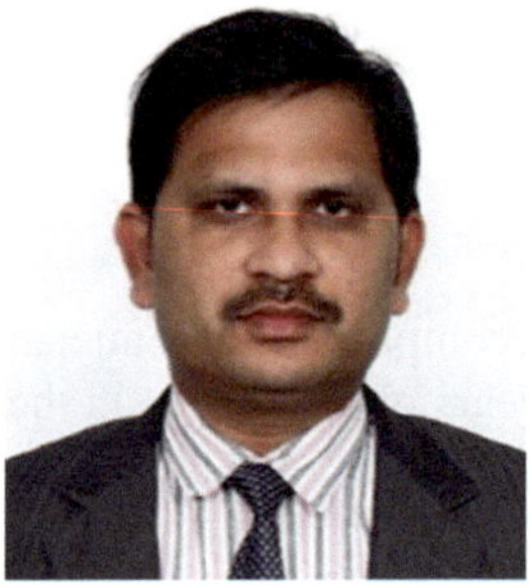

Sunil Gupta, Ph.D., M.Tech., B.E. has over more than 19 years of experience in teaching, research, and industry in the field of Computer Science and Engineering. Prior to joining UPES as a Professor, he has worked with, BML Munjal University, Delhi Technical Campus, IP University, Northern India Engineering College, IP University, IIMT, Baddi University of Emerging Science, IFTM University and Physical Laboratory. He is an active member of IEEE Society, Computer Society of India; Member, Computer Science Teacher Association; Life Member, International Association of Engineers; Member, International Association of Computer Science and Information Technology; and Member, Internet Society (ISOC). He has conducted various workshops, conferences, and FDP. He guides various students for research and project work. He is an authored 69 research papers, 6 patents, and 2 textbooks, namely *Cryptography and Network Security* and *Wireless Sensor Networks*. His academic interest includes Security, Cloud Computing, Big Data, Sensors, Wireless Networks, and Healthcare. He has successfully completed various research projects and consultancy from government and private organization like, Department of Science and Technology, Xcrino Business Solutions, and more. He has been regularly invited as a technical expert in different committees by both private and government organizations. He is an expert for recruiting faculty by different colleges affiliated to GGSIPU and has been nominated in JAC (Joint Assessment Committee) as a Technical Expert by GGSIPU to evaluate the functioning of various colleges (both Government and Private) affiliated to the same. He is a reviewer of international journals namely *Journal of Supercomputing*, published by Springer Netherlands, *International Journal of Wireless Networks* by Springer, *International Journal of Computer and*

Electrical Engineering, Singapore; and Member of Scientific Committee and Editorial Review Board on Engineering and Physical Sciences for World Academy of Science, Engineering and Technology and many more.

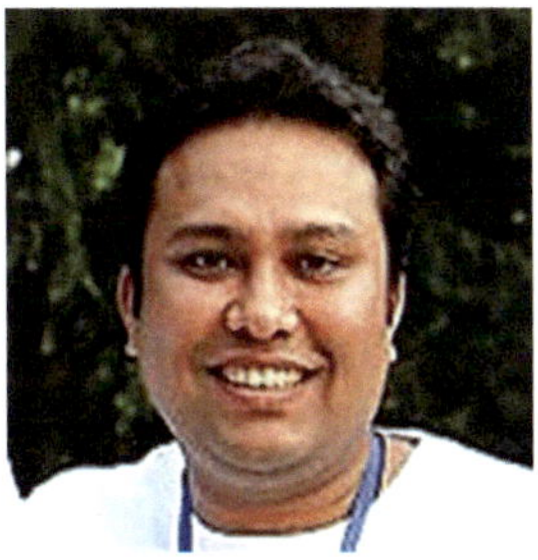

Abhishek Tyagi, Ph.D., M.Tech., B.Tech. has over 18 years of experience in teaching, research, and industry in the field of Nanotechnology, Biotechnology and Chemical Engineering. Currently he is working as Senior Formulation Scientist, Research and Development of Kings Flair Company; presently he is positioned in Melbourne, Victoria, Australia. He is responsible for the development of new chemical formulations for the novel biomaterials for healthcare products. Earlier, he worked as a research scholar in HKUST, Hong Kong, as an Assistant Professor in School of Biotechnology in IFTM University Moradabad, India, and SDCET Muzaffarnagar, India. He is an active member for the American Association for the Advancement of Science (AAAS), American Institute of Chemical Engineering (AIChE), and European Molecular Biology Laboratory (EMBL). As an aspirant researcher, he guided several ungraduated and postgraduate students for research projects and career guidance. He has conducted various workshops, conferences, and FDP programs. Dr. Tyagi has published more than 28 research articles and several conference articles. His research interest covers healthcare, nanotechnology, and bioengineering. As a faculty, he enjoyed teaching a wide range of subjects with their laboratory classes, for example, Nanotechnology, Biomaterials and Biomedical Engineering, Food Technology, etc. As a Healthcare Entrepreneur he has built, ideated, and validated his own business idea based on his Ph.D. research involving the development and commercialization of biosensors to be used in Bio-Pharmaceutical industry. He successfully graduated from the Hong Kong 3rd cohort and launched his start-up Aptacle Private Limited, Singapore. He is a reviewer of international journals of Springer Nature, Taylor & Francis Group, LLC, American Institute of Physics (AIP) Advances, Inderscience, PLOS One, and *Journal of Chemical Technology & Biotechnology*.

Chapter 1
Metaverse and Its Applications

1.1 Introduction: The Concept of Metaverse in Healthcare

The metaverse is a virtual, interconnected, immersive digital space beyond the physical world. It is basically a shared virtual space, usually accessed through the Internet, where one interacts with other people and digital objects in real time. In other words, it describes several technologies and platforms, including those of virtual reality, augmented reality, and mixed reality. The metaverse has recently gained much momentum because it could be used across a wide range of industries, from transforming healthcare to many more. Its relevance to healthcare can, therefore, be equated to creating those transformative approaches to the problems in the healthcare sector that have been sought for so long (Ullah et al. 2023).

1.1.1 Meta-Health: Relevance to Healthcare

Meta-Health defines this new frontier of the application of metaverse in healthcare. It is a new paradigm for delivering healthcare, education of professionals and patients, and patient engagement. Benefits and opportunities arise in several important ways, including but not limited to the following and described in Fig. 1.1:

- Telemedicine and Virtual Consultation: Metaverse would allow health professionals to consult from afar and care for patients in virtual space. This is quite useful, especially where the need exists to reach out to underserved or remote populations.
- Medical Training and Simulation: Metaverse will also be able to create hyper-realistic medical training and simulation training for health providers. Medical students and practitioners have the facility to practice their procedures, surgeries, and diagnostics in safety within a virtual setting.

S. Vyas et al., *Meta-Health*, https://doi.org/10.1007/978-981-96-5844-2_1

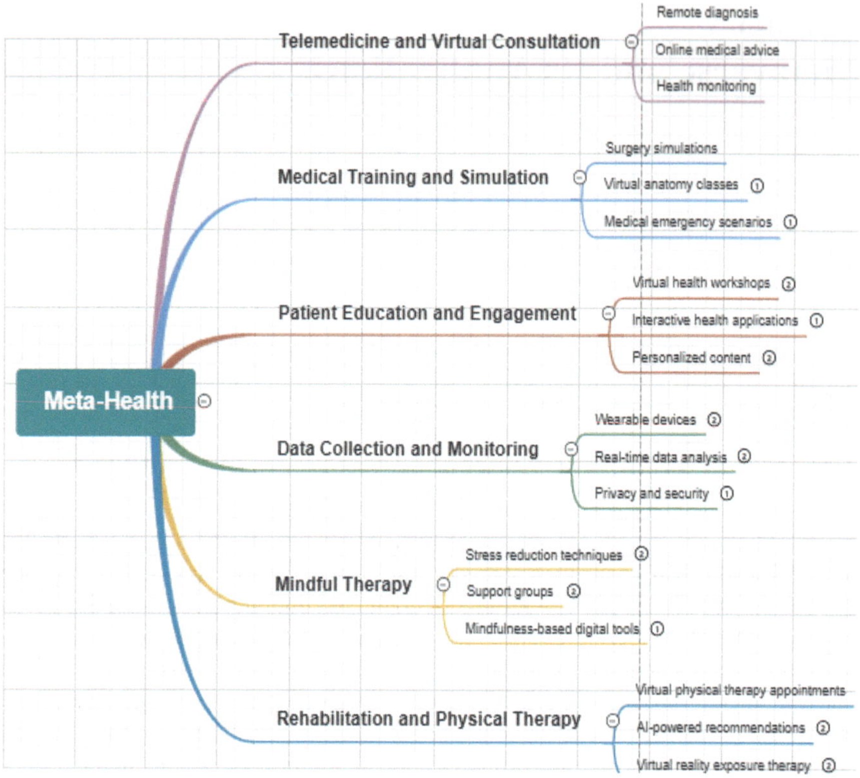

Fig. 1.1 Meta-Health benefits and opportunities

- Patient Education and Engagement: The virtual healthcare information, education, and support groups increase in the patient's understanding of their conditions and all options for treatment. Virtual communities like these can be employed for psychological support and fraternity.
- Data Collection and Monitoring: There is a range of wearables and sensors that could be used to monitor in real time the health of an individual, which can then seamlessly feed into the metaverse for ongoing, continuous monitoring. This will allow for the early detection of some diseases and permit personalized treatment.
- Mindful Therapy: A new virtual therapy and mental health provided in metaverse confirms that people have easier access to private spaces where they can receive support and treatment for various kinds of mental health conditions.
- Rehabilitation and Physical Therapy: The virtual space can also be used for physical rehabilitation and therapy. It will make training more interesting and encouraging for patients.

In other words, the metaverse in healthcare could democratize access to health services, improve patient outcomes, enhance residency training, and change the way healthcare is delivered and experienced (Houssein et al. 2024).

1.1.2 *Chapter Objectives*

This chapter should clearly and concisely introduce the concept of Meta-Health, defined as the metaverse for healthcare. It also needs to establish the relevance of the emerging field for possible impacts within the healthcare industry.

- The Application of Meta-Health: This chapter introduces the reader to the various applications of Meta-Health in Healthcare. It really deals with how virtual and augmented reality technologies, through the metaverse, can transform patient care and medical education, together with remote monitoring.
- Discussion of Challenges and Opportunities: The challenges and opportunities in the integration of metaverse into healthcare will be addressed, including major themes of privacy and security issues, ethics, and potential benefits related to improved access and quality of healthcare.
- Provide Real-World Examples: This chapter discusses real-world case studies and examples of successful implementations of Meta-Health. This would give examples of how healthcare organizations and professionals are already embracing virtual environments to improve the delivery and outcomes of healthcare.
- Discuss the Future of Meta-Health: The future prospects of Meta-Health are discussed here, emerging trends, technologies, and possible developments in personalized medicine, patient engagement, and healthcare innovation in the metaverse.

1.2 Overview: The Metaverse in Healthcare

The metaverse in health could be described as an immersive, virtual, completely interconnected digital environment outside traditional healthcare settings where a wide array of health-related activities, interactions, and services will be enabled. It is a virtual ecosystem through which patients, healthcare professionals, educators, and innovators will interact and gain access to healthcare resources, information, and experiences in newly developed technological ways.

The main elements of the metaverse in health are as follows and shown in Fig. 1.2a, b:

(a) Virtual Healthcare Environments: These are virtual and physically created digital environments simulating the real world of healthcare, which may include hospitals, clinics, and examination rooms. In these virtual healthcare environments, patients can receive virtual healthcare services and consultations. AR and VR in Healthcare: AR and VR have a great role in developing immersive and interactive experiences in healthcare. The key examples of their usage include training in medical treatment, patient education, pain management, and therapeutic interventions.

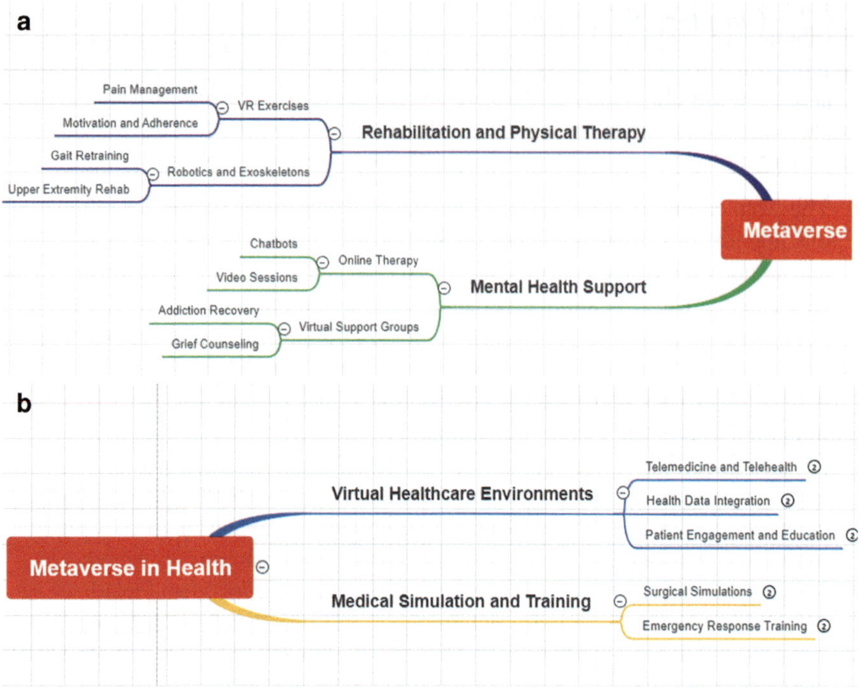

Fig. 1.2 (**a, b**) Elements of metaverse

(b) Telemedicine and Telehealth: Metaverse allows consultations and healthcare remotely. It virtually connects patients and providers. Certain telemedicine platforms in metaverse allow for real-time communication and diagnosis.
(c) Health Data Integration: Wearable devices and sensors monitor and collect data about the health of a patient in real time. Metaverse integrates this and presents valuable insights to healthcare professionals for diagnosis, monitoring treatment, etc.
(d) Patient Engagement and Education: Patients can access health information, education, and support groups without much hassle through the metaverse. Such a virtual setting creates unparalleled opportunities in engaging patients and enhancing health literacy.
(e) Medical Simulation and Training: Under this virtual environment, healthcare professionals and students can engage themselves in realistic simulations of medical training and practices that allow them to hone their skills and take better care of patients.
(f) Mental Health Support: Virtual therapy and mental health support services available on metaverse provide a discrete, fully immersive environment where one can share their mental health issues.

(g) Rehabilitation and Physical Therapy: Metaverse virtual environments are very useful for physical rehabilitation and therapy, since it can make patients more interested in exercises.

Health, better known as "Meta-Health," would be much enriched with these elements of metaverse, increasing access to quality healthcare services, enhancing medical education, and empowering patients to be more involved in their own health management. This also opens avenues to innovation and the creation of new, hopefully game-changing solutions that were previously thought impossible within the limitations of the physical world (Houssein et al. 2024).

1.2.1 Historical Background

Metaverse development and its application in the healthcare sector can be dated through several milestones. A historical overview of how the metaverse has evolved to influence healthcare:

- Early Virtual Worlds (1990s): In the 1990s, virtual worlds and online communities began taking shape. These included the likes of Second Life. While these early virtual spaces were not focused on healthcare originally, they indeed formed a basis for immersive online interactions.
- Introduction of Telemedicine: Telemedicine started to emerge around the early 2000s, which allowed for remote consultations between patients and providers. While still not counted as part of the metaverse at that time, it was a basic revolution in the delivery of health.
- Growth of Virtual Reality and Augmented Reality: Virtual reality and augmented reality technologies reached the final phase of advancement in the mid-2000s. These technologies have been employed in training for doctors and surgeons in the form of simulation surgeries.
- Virtual Health Communities Merge: The beginning of online health communities and support groups mushroomed in the 2010s. In this, patients were allowed to share experiences, advice, and seek company with others facing similar challenges in health.
- Virtual Reality in Medical Education: At this period of time, medical institutions and universities started the process of integrating the use of VR into the education and training of aspiring doctors; thus, allowing one to experience practice and surgery in a no-risk virtual environment.
- Telehealth Expansion (2020s): COVID-19 accelerated the introduction and utilization of telehealth and telemedicine. It was during this era that the next wave of metaverse integration with rapid transition toward remote health services was set into place.
- Metaverse Rise, 2020s: The concept of the metaverse finally entered widespread consciousness in the 2020s, hastened by tech giants and notably the concept of

Meta, formerly known as Facebook, in creating expansive virtual spaces. This recent focus on the metaverse aligns with the realization of its potential in health.
- Meta-Health and Healthcare Applications, 2020s–Present: Meta-Health. Now, every healthcare provider and innovator is looking into the applications of Meta-Health in virtual medical consultations, immersive training, mental health support, and data-driven healthcare experiences.
- Investment and Innovation: Increasing investments in metaverse-related healthcare technologies and startups have nurtured novel healthcare solutions that are starting to emerge within virtual environments.

Where the medical influence of the metaverse is concerned, historical evolution has reflected a gradual shift in embracing virtual and digital technologies to serve the manifold aspects of improvement in patient care, training, and experience. As the metaverse further expands and evolves, it will no doubt play a much larger role in shaping the future of healthcare by offering innovative solutions to new, emerging needs of both patients and healthcare professionals (Majumder and Dey 2024).

1.2.2 Virtual and Augmented Realities, Including Mixed Reality in Healthcare

Virtual reality, augmented reality, and mixed reality are representatives of transformative technologies that have found wide applications within the healthcare sector. Each of these immersive technologies has great unique capabilities, hence finding great significance in their role as a tool for patient care, medical training, and innovation in healthcare (Zhang et al. 2022). Let us discuss each VR, AR, and MR regarding healthcare below.

1.2.2.1 Virtual Reality in Healthcare

1. Medical Training and Simulation: These enable realistic and immersive simulations for medical professionals and students. Surgeons will be able to rehearse, in a virtual space, difficult procedures without putting their real patients at risk. The medical students can practice live in this virtual and safe place.
2. Pain Management and Distraction: It has also been used during painful procedures for the purpose of distracting the patient from pain, such as during changes of wound dressing or dental work. Immersive experiences reduce pain perception and anxiety.
3. Physical and Cognitive Rehabilitation: VR-based exercises are conducted in rehabilitative programs. In such, patients recuperating from injuries or surgeries can enjoy exercises that help them recover.
4. Exposure Therapy for Mental Health: VR is put to use in the treatment of mental health disorders, including phobias and PTSD. Patients get to come face to face

with their fears and learn to control these emotions in a virtual environment designed for safety.
5. Patient Education: Conditions and treatment options are elaborated with the help of VR to educate the patients. These could, therefore, be explained in a manner that is easy to understand and might be conveyed in a more interesting way.

1.2.2.2 Augmented Reality in Healthcare

1. Surgical Navigation: AR superimposes digital information onto the surgeon's field of vision intraoperatively. This can enable navigation with high precision and decrease the risk of complications.
2. Medical Imagining: AR enhances the ability to view, touch, and interact with three-dimensional medical images for diagnostics and a better understanding. This permits surgeons to "see through" a patient's body in order to plan procedures.
3. Remote Assistance: Such AR can enable an expert at another location to guide residents or practitioners in real time. Surgeons operating may wear AR glasses transmitting their field of view for interaction by remote specialists.
4. Anatomical Visualization: AR apps are being developed and made available to both medical students and healthcare professionals for viewing, simulating, and interacting with anatomical models for further understanding of the human body.

1.2.2.3 Mixed Reality (MR) in Healthcare

1. Holographic Displays: MR headsets, like those from Microsoft HoloLens, will project holographic images into the field of vision of users. The displays can be used for anatomical visualization, surgical planning, and education.
2. Remote Collaboration: MR allows the collaboration of healthcare professionals on work even when they are kept apart, physically. Specialists will have the capability to share diagnoses and treatment plans with one another through holographic images.
3. Rehabilitation and Physical Therapy: MR will be able to make interactive and engaging rehabilitation exercises for patients that will enhance their recovery by making them more motivated.
4. Telemedicine and Consultations: MR could allow for a much more immersive and interactive telehealth experience by overlaying medical information onto the environment of a patient to inform diagnostics and consultations remotely.

1.3 Applications of the Metaverse in Healthcare

Applications of the metaverse to healthcare, a term popularly referred to as "Meta-Health," are incredibly varied and have the potential to cause revolutionary changes in many aspects of the healthcare industry (Bhatia and Joshi 2023). Following is some of the key applications of the metaverse in healthcare.

1.3.1 Telemedicine and Virtual Healthcare Services

Some of the most prominent and transformational uses of the metaverse in healthcare surround telemedicine and virtual health services. Virtual healthcare delivery models offer medical consultations, diagnosis, treatment, and support to patients through virtual environments. Here is how the metaverse is changing telemedicine and virtual healthcare service provision.

Virtual Consultations: Patients seek healthcare services from the comfort of their homes. People residing in remote or under-resourced regions do not have to necessarily visit a hospital or clinic for medical consultations.

- Convenience: Virtual consultations will eliminate the need to make physical visits to clinics. This saves time and consequently lessens burdens on health facilities. Patients can schedule their appointments at any time that best suits them.
- Specialized Care: Patients will be able to consult with any specialist in the world, ensuring high-level specialized medical care.

1.3.1.1 Realistic Healthcare Environments

- Immersive Clinics: Virtual healthcare can be designed with virtual clinics to give the patient a realistic experience of being inside a clinic while consulting with specialists.
- Specialized Virtual Clinics: Depending on a patient's condition or need, they should be given the opportunity to be handled or treated by a virtual clinic that caters to that particular need.

1.3.1.2 Improved Doctor-Patient Interaction

- Visualization: Doctors can leverage interactive 3D models, graphs, and visualizations in metaverse for better explanations of medical conditions and treatment plans to the patients.

- Nonverbal Communication: VR is capable of capturing nonverbal cues. The quality of doctor-patient interactions becomes much superior compared to traditional telehealth solutions.

1.3.1.3 Remote Monitoring and Data Integration

- Wearable Devices: Patients use wearable health monitoring devices connected to virtual healthcare environments and transmit real-time health data.
- Data Integration: Integration of data from various sources in support of diagnosis, treatment, and prevention.

1.3.1.4 Pharmacy and Medication Management

- Virtual Pharmacies: It will be possible to order medicines through virtual pharmacies within the metaverse so that there will be no delay in access to a prescription.
- Medication Reminders: Virtual healthcare environments remind one when medications are due and support the patient in medication adherence.

1.3.1.5 Mental Health and Therapy Services

- Virtual Therapy: Patients with issues regarding mental health can access virtual therapy sessions and counseling in a very private immersive environment.
- Support Groups: The virtual support groups for mental health conditions make one feel part of the community with peer support.

1.3.1.6 Emergencies and Triage

- Virtual Emergency Rooms: During emergencies, patients will be treated No in the virtual emergency room, which will triage and assess the patient for further treatment in the physical facility.

1.3.1.7 Multiplayer Healthcare Consultations

- Family or Caregiver Participation: Virtual consultations may include multiple participants, including family or caregivers, to support the patient or to discuss decisions about the care being provided to the patient.

1.3.2 *Medical Training and Education in Virtual Environments*

Training and education are one of the novel applications of the metaverse in healthcare. Immersive technologies ensure a realistic and interactive learning environment for health professionals and students alike (Pieterse et al. 2023). The following shows how metaverse is revolutionizing medical training and education:

1.3.2.1 Surgery Simulations

- Realistic Procedures: The virtual environment lets the surgeon practice in high fidelity and realism.
- Skill Development: Surgeons practice skills, improve hand-eye coordination, and get accustomed to new surgical instruments and their use techniques.

1.3.2.2 Anatomy and Physiology Education

- Interactive 3D Models: The virtual environment provides three-dimensional models of the human body for in-depth studies of anatomy and physiology.
- Dissection Simulations: Students will be able to virtually perform the dissection of organs and tissues internally and thus deeply study human anatomy without the need to use actual cadavers.

1.3.2.3 Medical Diagnosis and Decision-Making

- Clinical Scenarios: Virtual patients with different pathologies and symptoms offer the student a chance to study and practice their diagnostic skills and also sharpen clinical judgment.
- Treatment Planning: The student can design and implement a treatment plan, including the prescription of medication and surgical intervention in virtual environments.

1.3.2.4 Emergency Medicine Training

- Simulated Emergencies: Healthcare professionals can practice for high-stress situations using virtual emergencies like trauma or cardiac arrest.
- Team-Based Training: Interdisciplinary healthcare teams could practice coordination and communication in simulated emergencies.

1.3.2.5 Distance Learning and Collaboration

- Anywhere Access: Medical virtual training can be accessed anywhere, hence reducing the need for a physical presence within the training facilities.
- Global Collaboration: In the metaverse, students and professionals at different ends of the globe can get connected discussing cases and projects on research.

1.3.2.6 Continuing Medical Education CME

- Virtual CME Conferences: Health professionals attend virtual CME conferences, workshops, and seminars to stay updated about the latest medical advances and research.

1.3.2.7 Patient Interaction and Communication Skills

- Practice of Bedside Manner: Medical students are allowed to practice talking with patients, showing empathy, and practicing bedside manners in the virtual encounters.
- Cultural Competency: A virtual environment can be used to simulate interactions with patients coming from a diverse set of cultural backgrounds, enhancing cultural competency.

1.3.2.8 Ethical Dilemma Scenarios

Ethics Training

- Virtual scenarios place medical professionals in ethical dilemmas where practice in ethics decision-making and critical thinking is needed.

Interdisciplinary Education

- Collaborative Learning: Students in health professions of medicine, nursing, and pharmacy will learn through virtual interdisciplinary learning teams on solving complex healthcare cases.

Feedback and Assessment

- Immediate Feedback: The virtual simulations will be offering instantaneous feedback on performance to help learners recognize where their improvement lies.

1.3.2.9 Specialized Curricula

- Subspecialty Training: Specialized training programs, like interventional radiology or robotic surgery training, may also be made available in the virtual environment.
- Medically relevant education and training, taking place in virtual environments called metaverse, will facilitate improvements in learning outcomes, enhance the acquisition of better skills, and thus better prepare health workers for real-life clinical practice. Such applications have added value when working on problems related to limited access to clinical experience and to continuous professional development.

1.3.3 Virtual Therapy and Mental Health Support

Mental health support and virtual therapy will open an entire new frontier in the metaverse. Applications make use of immersive digital environments in a manner such that mental health services and support become accessible, private, and effective for all people. Here is how virtual therapy and mental health support make a difference (Chen et al. 2023).

1.3.3.1 Accessible and Convenient Counseling

- Remote Access: Virtual therapy has the potential to provide mental health access from anywhere and thereby transcend geography, thus improving access in rural or underserved areas.
- Flexible Scheduling: Patients are able to schedule therapy sessions at times most opportunely coinciding with their schedules; thus, there is greater convenience associated with a reduction in potential barriers to help-seeking.

1.3.3.2 Privacy and Anonymity

- Privacy: Most sessions of virtual therapies are kept private and confidential in nature to keep the patient's identity private.
- Less Stigma: There is little stigma associated with virtual therapy, since individuals can participate from their house without feeling judged for entering a clinic.

1.3.3.3 Different Modalities of Care

- Cognitive Behavioral Therapy: Virtual platforms provide evidence-based treatments such as CBT, which enable clients to manage a range of mental health conditions.
- Exposure Therapy: The use of virtual environments for exposure therapy in treating phobias, PTSD, and anxiety disorders lets patients gradually be exposed to their phobic elements in a compassionate, controlled, and highly immersive setting.
- Mindfulness and Relaxation: Such VR experiences can be utilized in conducting or leading patients through mindfulness and relaxation activities that help reduce stress and manage their symptoms.

1.3.3.4 Support for Specific Populations

- Veterans: Virtual therapy is one way of providing mental health support for veterans, especially to those who suffer from trauma and PTSD.
- Children and Adolescents: Virtual therapy platforms are designed to entertain younger populations. Therapy will be even more interactive and fun for children and teenagers.

1.3.3.5 Therapist-Patient Interaction

- Emotion Recognition: Virtual therapy platforms can include face expression and emotion recognition to let the therapist identify the emotional states of their patients during sessions.
- Body Language: VR can track body language and gestures, thus enabling therapists to make out more about the well-being of their patients.

1.3.3.6 Group Therapy and Support Groups

- e-Virtual Support Communities: The patients will be allowed to participate in virtual support groups and communities of others experiencing similar mental health challenges for a sense of belonging and being supported.

1.3.3.7 Decreasing Barriers to Access

- Reduced Wait Times: Virtual therapy will reduce the waiting period to access mental health services and, therefore, respond to a need that is usually so pressing for timely care.
- More Providers Available: Virtual therapy platforms increase the availability of mental health professionals, which enables more patients to get well on time.

1.3.3.8 Original Therapeutic Tools

- Biofeedback: The virtual environment can include mechanisms for biofeedback that allow patients to learn how to manage physiological responses associated with stress and anxiety.
- VRET or Virtual Reality Exposure Therapy: This involves a patient in a virtual scenario, relevant to their specific phobias or trauma. The process helps the patients during desensitization and cure.

This is where virtual therapy and mental health support within the metaverse are bridging gaps in service delivery, affording options to individuals in which they can seek help effectively and conveniently to manage their mental health and improve their general well-being. The applications are becoming increasingly important, particularly in addressing the rising demand for mental health services across the globe.

1.4 Remote Monitoring and Data Collection

Remote monitoring and data collection in the metaverse are crucial parts of modern healthcare and, therefore, depend on new digital technologies that enable the monitoring of the health of a patient and the collection of real-time data to enhance healthcare delivery. The following describe how does this remote monitoring and data collection change healthcare in the metaverse.

1.4.1 Wearable Devices and Sensors

- Continuous Health Tracking: Patients may wear various wearable devices, from smartwatches and fitness trackers, equipped with sensors for heart rate, blood pressure, and sleep pattern monitoring.
- Chronic Disease Management: It is of particular importance in chronic conditions like diabetes, wherein this remote monitoring can also measure glucose continuously and collect continuous data.

1.4.2 Virtual Care Platform Integration

- Data Visualization: Remote monitoring data can be integrated into the virtual health environment to enable a patient, as well as healthcare professionals, to view health trends and make appropriate decisions.

- Real-Time Alerts: Virtual health environments can provide real-time alerts and notifications regarding data received from wearable devices, thus making sure that timely interventions are not missed.

1.4.3 Telehealth and Virtual Consultations

- Data-Driven Consultation: Remote monitoring data enhances the quality of virtual consultations in that it provides updates to healthcare professionals about patients.
- Individualized Care Plans: Healthcare professionals can develop treatment plans and interventions based on individual needs.

1.4.4 Chronic Disease Management

- Medication Adherence: Virtual reminders and alerts can be used to facilitate the process, which is considered highly imperative for dealing with chronic diseases.
- Early Detection: Remote monitoring may allow early detentions in health indicators that would lead to timely changes in treatment plans and complications prevention.

1.4.5 Patient Engagement

- Empowerment: Remote monitoring has empowered patients to be more concerned with their health by understanding daily habits, physical activity, and changes in health metrics.
- Gamification: Virtual healthcare environments can utilize concepts of gamification in encouraging health and wellness activities, thereby making remote monitoring and data collection an exciting and engaging activity for the patients.

1.4.6 Mental Health Monitoring

- Stress and Mood Tracking: Wearables can track surges related to stress levels and mood. This would be a mine of information on mental health assessment and treatment.
- Therapist Insights: With remote monitoring, it will be easy for mental health specialists to understand their patients' feelings between sessions of therapy.

1.4.7 Data Privacy and Security

- Secure Data Transmission: Data from wearable devices and sensors are securely transmitted to virtual healthcare environments, maintaining patient privacy and protecting their data.
- Compliance with HIPAA: Virtual health platforms follow all major healthcare data privacy regulations, such as HIPAA, for keeping data confidential.

1.4.8 Research and Population Health

- Data Aggregation: Aggregated remote monitoring data from a large population could provide support for medical research, epidemiological studies, and public health initiatives. The next level of analytics can find trends and patterns in the health data to allow predictive modeling and proactive healthcare interventions.
- Remote monitoring and data collection in the metaverse are highly instrumental for proactive, personalized healthcare. Such applications will afford, through the capabilities of digital technologies, improved patient outcomes, more engagement of patients in their care, and greater efficiency in healthcare delivery.

1.5 Patient Engagement and Rehabilitation in the Metaverse

Patient engagement and rehabilitation in the metaverse create new dimensions for improvements in quality and effectiveness of rehabilitation programs. These applications employ immersive virtual environments that inspire and support patients on their journeys to recovery. Here is how patient engagement and rehabilitation in the metaverse are making the difference (Suh et al. 2023).

1.5.1 Gamified Rehabilitation Exercises

1. Engaging Activities: Rehabilitation exercises can be made interactive and gamified in virtual environments and hence quite enjoyable on the part of the patient.
2. Motivation: Rewards, challenges, and progress tracking are some of the gamification elements that motivate patients to adhere to their rehabilitation routines for better results.
3. Customized Rehabilitation Programs: Draw customized programs with the use of a virtual rehabilitation platform in accordance with the needs and conditions of every single patient, which means catching up on targeted therapy.

4. Progress Tracking: This data recorded in the metaverse can be used to track progress by both patients and health providers. All this will enable necessary amendments in rehabilitation processes.
5. Accessible Care: The access to metaverse will make the rehabilitation services available for remote application to the patients, reducing frequent face-to-face visits.
6. Continuous Support: The virtual environment will facilitate the communications and support continuously from the professional to ensure that feedback on time and changes are affected in rehabilitation programs.

1.5.2 Physical Rehabilitation

1. Range of Motion Exercises (ROM) Exercises: VR can guide the patients through exercises to enhance joint flexibility and mobility.
2. Balance and Coordination: Virtual environments challenge patients by making them exercise for balance and coordination to avoid falls and other injuries.

1.5.3 Cognitive Rehabilitation

1. Brain Training Games: Virtual platforms boast cognitive exercises and games supportive for patients in recovery either from brain injuries or impairments of cognition.
2. Improvement of Memory: Metaverse-based rehabilitation can also include engagement in activities aimed at improving memory among patients with cognitively related challenges in memory.

1.5.4 Virtual Physical Therapy Sessions

1. Live Feedback: A session of virtual therapy can be utilized to provide instant feedback about the form and improvement made by patients from physical therapists.
2. Demonstration: Exercises and proper techniques can be demonstrated with the help of virtual therapists in ways that are easy for patients to understand.

1.5.5 Interactive Virtual Environments

1. Scenic Settings: Virtual rehabilitation settings have the capability to transport patients to scenic locations. This, in turn, provides the visual and audio stimuli that make the therapy process more enjoyable.
2. Exploration and Adventure: Gamified rehabilitation environments encourage patients to explore and complete the challenges, hence participating in physical activities.

1.5.6 Support for Specific Conditions

1. Orthopedic Rehabilitation: Patients after joint replacements, fractures, or orthopedic surgeries may undergo focused exercises in virtual rehabilitation.
2. Stroke Recovery: A virtual environment can provide specified exercises that will help regain motor skills lost due to stroke.

1.5.7 Mental Health Support in Rehabilitation

1. Stress Reduction: The use of VR in creating soothing and relaxing environments can help reduce stress and be helpful for mental well-being during rehabilitation.
2. Integrating Mental Health: Such rehabilitation programs may integrate modules that address the psychological components of recovery, including anxiety and depression.

1.5.8 Social Support and Collaboration

1. Virtual Support Groups: Being part of virtual support groups dealing with rehabilitation may allow patients to feel like they belong and have something in common.
2. Engaging the Caregiver: Virtual worlds can afford opportunities for caregivers to be involved in the rehabilitation of their loved ones.

Patient-centered engagement in and rehabilitation within the metaverse are highly advanced technological ways of recovery, thus allowing better compliance with the rehabilitation process and favorable outcomes in overall well-being. Applications to specific scenarios are particularly useful in long-term rehabilitation and in patients with various levels of mobility.

1.6 Challenges and Opportunities

The integration of the metaverse in healthcare would have several applications, including but not limited to Meta-Health, virtual therapy, remote monitoring, and rehabilitation. Each of these areas carries challenges and opportunities. What follows is some balancing regarding the key challenges and opportunities with respect to using the metaverse for healthcare (Rawal et al. 2022).

1.6.1 Challenges

(a) Digital Divide: The majority cannot access the required technology or connectivity to be able to avail of virtual healthcare services, creating disparities in healthcare access.
(b) Privacy and Security: Virtual healthcare environments are those that are under strict law, such as HIPAA, protecting patient information but also targets for cyberattacks.
(c) Ethics: There are a host of other ethical issues involved with patient consent, ownership of data, and addiction or abuse associated with virtual environments.
(d) Interoperability: What different virtual healthcare platforms and electronic health records can be interoperable to share data remains a technical challenge.
(e) Quality Assurance: The standards would continually need to be updated concerning the quality of care and valid medical training that is given out in virtual environments.
(f) Digital Fatigue: Too much time spent in virtual life may give way to digital fatigue with plausible adverse effects on mental health.
(g) Regulatory Hurdles: Regulations and policies about healthcare are bound to lag and need urgent updating and adapting to the metaverse.

These are better overcome through collaboration between health organizations, technology companies, policymakers, and patient advocacy groups. Implantation of the metaverse in healthcare also requires a commitment toward privacy, security, ethics, and equity so that benefits can be achieved without loss of patient well-being and safety as mentioned in Fig. 1.3.

1.6.2 Opportunities

This, of course, will include applications involving the use of Meta-Health, virtual therapy, remote monitoring, and rehabilitation. Several opportunities, inclusive but not limited to those above, exist that can be greatly instrumental in improving

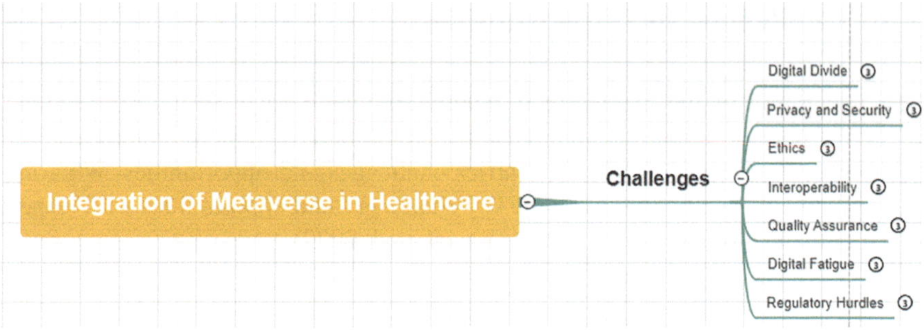

Fig. 1.3 Challenges in integration of metaverse with healthcare

healthcare delivery and patient outcomes (Rawal et al. 2022). Key opportunities will include the following:

(a) Improved Access to Care: The metaverse will break down barriers and allow populations that are remote or underserved to access healthcare services and reduce disparities in healthcare.
(b) Patient-Centric Care: The virtual healthcare environment can be a strong tool for enabling patients to play an active role in their own care by acquiring, processing, and understanding basic health information and making informed decisions regarding their health and well-being.
(c) Improved Engagement and Adherence: Immersive and engaging virtual healthcare experiences can motivate patients toward treatment plan adherence and result in improved health outcomes of better quality, especially in the management of chronic diseases and rehabilitation.
(d) Personalized Medicine: It also brings a great deal of extended patient data and thereby the capability to make personalized treatment plans and interventions specific to the need and condition of the individual patient. This would also enable remote monitoring and facilitate early detection of:
(e) The ability to use continuous monitoring from a distance allows the establishment of health problems in their early stages, thus enabling interventions in time. This enables the prevention of further diseases.
(f) Cost Efficiency: The use of virtual healthcare may reduce the cost associated with maintaining physical infrastructure and administrative processes. It makes healthcare more cost-effective.
(g) Global Collaboration: This could also mean that medical professionals, researchers, and patients from around the world could collaborate in virtual worlds and make the process of medical research and innovation more efficient. To this regard:
(h) Personalization: Healthcare in the metaverse will be customized to meet the specific needs and preferences of individual patients, making the treatment much more personalized.

(i) Mental Health Support: As an increasing number of people suffer from mental health problems, scaling virtual treatment or mental health support faces lower barriers in terms of both accessibility and stigma.
(j) Advanced Rehabilitation: Virtual rehabilitation programs improve patients' motivation and outcomes, especially for those cases that require long-term and chronic treatments, and this is feasible remotely.
(k) Public Health Initiatives: The metaverse would enable public health campaigns, health education, and emergency preparedness to take place and improve community health status.
(l) Data-Driven Insights: Remote monitoring and data collecting provide frontline beneficial datasets for healthcare analytics and build predictive modeling and evidence-based decision-making.
(m) Innovative Training: Virtual simulation will also lead to experiential advanced training and skill development of healthcare professionals, making them even safer and more competent medical practitioners.
(n) Crisis Response: Virtual healthcare can be quickly set up in crises situations and provide some necessary care and supplies to the affected population.
(o) Reduced Stigma: The virtual healthcare services may reduce the stigma associated with seeking help regarding mental health issues and make it more acceptable and accessible.
(p) Support for Special Populations: This might also be adapted to accommodate veterans' needs, children, and persons with disabilities.

For this, effective exploitation requires collaboration between healthcare providers, technology companies, regulators, and patients to realize all the benefits of the metaverse in health while challenges are taken into consideration, together with patients' privacy, safety, and ethics.

1.7 Case Studies and Real-World Examples

1.7.1 VR for Pain Management

The Cedars-Sinai Medical Center in Los Angeles, California, uses virtual reality technology to help manage pain in hospitalized patients. Such patients can be taken through relaxing virtual environments that help them reduce their perception of pain and anxiety. This practice reduces the use of opioids and offers a greater comfort level for ailing individuals (Liu and Dong 2016).

Outcome: VR-based pain management has been successful in a wide range of healthcare areas and thus finds its application as a non-pharmacological substitute in pain management.

1.7.2 Virtual Reality Exposure Therapy (VRET) for Phobia

Researchers and therapists are applying the use of VR in treating specific phobia situations such as flying, heights, or spiders. Patients are exposed to some form of phobia while in a controlled virtual state in small doses that will assist them in facing and controlling their anxiety attack.

Impact: VRET has been proven successful in desensitizing the patients from their phobias and is currently a valued tool in mental health therapy.

1.7.3 Virtual Surgical Training Environments

Medical institutions like Stanford University and the Cleveland Clinic are using VR and AR technology on their respective virtual platforms for surgical training. Surgeries can be practiced in a fully immersive virtual environment without risking real lives.

Impact: VR as a platform for surgical training harbors better surgical skills, fewer errors, and hence better patient outcomes.

1.7.4 VR for Physical Rehabilitation

Virtual reality is now being included in various physical therapy clinics and rehabilitation centers; it enables patients in recovery from injuries or surgeries to engage in exercises using VR methods that are much more enjoyable and motivating for them.

Impact: This might improve patient compliance and further reduce recovery time, which would improve physical therapy outcomes using VR.

1.7.5 Virtual Support Groups for Mental Health

Case Study: Virtual support groups and therapy sessions have been developed for people with mental health problems by different organizations, particularly in the COVID-19 pandemic. The users of these groups develop a sense of belongingness and peer relationships.

Impact: The accessibility of mental health services through virtual support groups lessens the loneliness of the participants of such groups (Liu and Dong 2016).

1.7.6 Future Prospect of Meta-Health

In this regard, the future possibilities of Meta-Health have emerged as a transformational paradigm in the realm of healthcare. The traction, which is represented by the fusion between metaverse, and healthcare is enormous, though little more than a conceptual tapestry woven through the emerging possibilities. On this picturesque canvas, we are going to visualize the following theoretical vistas (https://www.pwc.com/m1/en/industries/healthcare/the-future-of-healthcare-in-the-metaverse.html):

- Immersive telemedicine worlds-the transformation of the world into an immersive telehealth experience beyond the confines of screen and wire. Patients will navigate virtual corridors to meet holographic physicians; their avatars play host to all that medical learning. The promise herein is holistic, accessible, interrelated health services across theoretical immersivity's that bridge geographic divides.
- Theoretically, the Holo-Healers and Digital Companions materialize as AI-driven holographic healers and digital companions that stand in companionship on the journey of man through his healthcare. These sentient constructs, smitten with machine learning prowess, mete out emotional support, recommendations for treatments, and companionship in times of need.
- Neural-Link Interfaces: The neural-link interfaces of the near future will mediate direct-brain interaction with the metaverse. Patients will simply think about virtual health interfaces that pop up, and they will access medical data, therapies, and diagnostics in virtual real time. Such neural pathways make it difficult to establish what part is the human mind and what part is the virtual world.
- Quantum Data Vaults: Data security has turned out to be of prime importance; thus, the theoretical quantum data vaults have come into being as strongholds of health information impregnable. Quantum encryption keys guard patient information and ensure complete security with absolute privacy in the virtual space.
- Genetic Exploration with Digital Laboratories: Deep insights into the human genome in their theoretical virtual laboratories in the metaverse can be created with virtual precision in taking apart the intricacies of the genetic code. Moving along this virtual frontier, researchers can understand the working of any disease etiology faster and boost drug discovery with personalized medicine.
- Pandemic Palisades: The metaverse creates theoretical pandemic palisades in the shadow of pandemics. These virtual bulwarks allow for the quickest response and thus enable virtual epidemiology and crisis control. People and health professionals will cluster in protected spaces to stop contagion and spread wisdom to sufferers.
- The Ethereal Healer's Oath: The theoretical Ethereal Healer's Oath is an equivalent of the Hippocratic Oath in a virtual metaverse and binds healers to principles of empathy, beneficence, and ethical stewardship. The oath defines that health professionals should utilize their digital powers for the benefit of humans by protecting the sacred trust between a patient and their healer.

- Theoretically speaking, there is room for conceptual frameworks of global harmonization and ethical consensus when the boundaries of Meta-Health expand. It is here that nations and entities begin to collect and come to a consensus on one single page regarding standards of virtual health, which ensures complete access to codes of ethics and the free flow of knowledge across the borders.
- Transcendental Well-being: Theoretical Meta-Health surpasses the physical sphere and creates an integrated area for health. Patients oversee and manage their journey of transition through spiritual oases in the metaverse and improve states of health and calm by the powers of mindfulness, meditation, and holistic rehabilitation.
- Meta-epistemology: Theoretically, meta-epistemology becomes a branch of the study of knowledge, truth, and wisdom within Meta-Health. Theoreticians thus explore the conceptual footing of this new field to make sense of the ontological and epistemological aspects of healthcare in the metaverse.

In this tapestry of theory, the prospects of Meta-Health have barely crystallized, but the potential to redefine even the very core of health is undeniably deep. As much as these theoretical vistas are but whispers from the horizon, they beckon us toward a future in which the very boundaries of the conceivable dissolve into a novel era of healthcare—a realm in which the ethereal and the empirical come together to tender the betterment of humanity.

1.8 Conclusion

The metaverse, integrated into healthcare, launches light on a transformative frontier—a promise in the contours of healthcare delivery and patient experiences. This conceptual convergence joins bleeding-edge technologies like virtual and augmented reality with the core mission of healthcare into a new frontier of accessibility, interaction of patients, data-driven insight, and innovating training in medicine. But while treading the path of Meta-Health opens up many new vistas, it equally points to major challenges: everything from data privacy concerns to the imperative of ethical considerations requires sensitive navigation and adaptation at a regulatory level. Though this new frontier remains beset on all sides with uncertainties, the beacon that is Meta-Health beckons brightly to take healthcare across its traditional boundaries into a future wherein healthcare will no longer be confined to the physical but stretches into the endless expanses of the metaverse, promising a health renaissance—the ethereal married to the empirical in a harmonious union aimed at bettering the human condition.

References

Bhatia B, Joshi S (2023) Applications of metaverse in the healthcare industry. In: 2023 international conference on innovative data communication technologies and application (ICIDCA), Uttarakhand, India, pp 344–350. https://doi.org/10.1109/ICIDCA56705.2023.10099897

Chen WC, Chan HY, Sung YH et al (2023) Therapists' practical implementation and preparation of online counseling in the post-pandemic era. Curr Psychol 42:30548–30560. https://doi.org/10.1007/s12144-023-04614-0

Houssein EH, Saber E, Ali AA et al (2024) Integrating metaheuristics and artificial intelligence for healthcare: basics, challenging and future directions. Artif Intell Rev 57:205. https://doi.org/10.1007/s10462-024-10822-2

Liu ZJ, Dong H (2016) Virtual reality technology for pain management. In: Langdon P, Lazar J, Heylighen A, Dong H (eds) Designing around people. Springer, Cham. https://doi.org/10.1007/978-3-319-29498-8_8

Majumder S, Dey N (2024) Application of metaverse services to the healthcare industry. In: Metaverse for industry 5.0, SpringerBriefs in applied sciences and technology. Springer, Singapore. https://doi.org/10.1007/978-981-97-2455-0_15

Pieterse AD, Hierck BP, de Jong PGM et al (2023) User experiences of medical students with 360-degree virtual reality applications to prepare them for the clerkships. Virtual Reality 27:1381–1389. https://doi.org/10.1007/s10055-022-00731-6

Rawal BS, Ahmadand S, Mentges A, Fadli S (2022) Opportunities and challenges in metaverse the rise of digital universe. In: Zhang LJ (ed) Metaverse—METAVERSE 2022, Lecture notes in computer science, vol 13737. Springer, Cham. https://doi.org/10.1007/978-3-031-23518-4_1

Suh I, McKinney T, Siu K-C (2023) Current perspective of metaverse application in medical education, research and patient care. Virtual Worlds 2:115–128. https://doi.org/10.3390/virtualworlds2020007

Ullah H, Manickam S, Obaidat M, Laghari SUA, Uddin M (2023) Exploring the potential of metaverse technology in healthcare: applications, challenges, and future directions. IEEE Access 11:69686–69707. https://doi.org/10.1109/ACCESS.2023.3286696

Zhang J, Yu N, Wang B et al (2022) Trends in the use of augmented reality, virtual reality, and mixed reality in surgical research: a global bibliometric and visualized analysis. Indian J Surg 84(Suppl 1):52–69. https://doi.org/10.1007/s12262-021-03243-w

Chapter 2
Revolution of Healthcare Industry

2.1 Introduction

The healthcare world continues to evolve at rapid paces with the integration of digital technologies, increased attention to personalized medicine, and shifting paradigms to patient-centered care at the core of such revolution. Actually, this has pulled apart traditional ways in which healthcare is provided, managed, or even experienced. While genomics and pharmacogenomics forge ahead, personalized medicine certainly outshines general approaches to treatment, which have been the dominant trait of traditional medicine by having treatments designed for resonance with a person's specific genetic makeup in consideration for more effective and targeted therapies. The initiation of big data and AI in healthcare is remodeling diagnostics, predictive analytics, and drug development into insights previously unseen, thereby enhancing decision-making. With the patient base increasingly aware and involved, the focus shifts to patient-centered care. The digital solutions enable improved education, shared decision-making, and management of chronic diseases. At the same time as this rapid progress, equally significant challenges include data privacy, ethical considerations related to AI, and an approach to inequities in healthcare. This chapter focuses on each of these critical aspects of the ongoing revolution in the healthcare industry, what are the forces driving change, how changes in the healthcare industry affect patients and providers, and future directions that continue to reshape the industry.

2.2 Overview of the Healthcare Industry's Transformation

All these have combined in a series of technological changes, changing patient expectations, and systemic changes in healthcare delivery that have transformed the healthcare industry in the last few decades. Significant to this transformation has

S. Vyas et al., *Meta-Health*, https://doi.org/10.1007/978-981-96-5844-2_2

been the integration of digital technologies, which has fundamentally changed how healthcare services are provided, managed, and accessed. EHR replaced the paper-based system, which manages data much more effectively and, because of this management, allows for better coordination of care and raises the level of accuracy in patient records. Telemedicine broadens access to health services due to which patients can now receive consulting services from medical professionals from the comfort of their homes, thus bridging the gap in care after hospital discharge, especially in areas that have a shortage of providers or are rural.

Another deep modification is represented by the passage from a one-size-fits-all approach to personalized medicine, that is, treatment according to one's own genetic background, lifestyle, and environmental exposures. Such a step forward was made possible to the advances in genomics and pharmacogenomics that allow targeted therapies and a more specific treatment planning to improve patient outcomes and reduce side effects.

Analytics and AI provided a new wave in the healthcare field with tools for predictive analytics, advanced diagnostics, and optimized treatment strategies. Big data makes it possible to analyze large volumes of health information for patterns and trends that inform clinical decisions and improve patient care. Artificial intelligence and machine learning algorithms support diagnosis of diseases, predict the outcomes of patients, and personalize treatments to move healthcare into more data-driven and precise medicine.

The other fundamental transformation in the industry has been to focus on the patient-centered aspect of care. In this respect, patients are becoming increasingly engaged in their healthcare through various digital tools, enabling access to health information, shared decision-making, and the management of conditions. All this puts considerable emphasis on aligning health services with patient preferences and needs to ultimately improve the experience and outcomes.

Despite such development, transition of healthcare faces challenges on various fronts: data privacy and security, ethics of AI, and still-more healthcare disparities ensure that benefits arising out of these developments are distributed equitably. Therefore, striking a balance between technological advancements with these considerations must be done in order to move towards efficiency, effectiveness, and greater inclusiveness in healthcare (Hermes et al. 2020).

2.2.1 Key Drivers of Change

This sets up various factors that have driven this transformation in the health sector and helped shape the healthcare industry into an increasingly innovative, efficient, and responsive system. These include technological advancement, policy reforms, evolving expectations of the patient, and the pursuit of improved health outcomes.

2.2.1.1 Technological Advancements

- Digital Health Technologies: EHRs and other health information systems have been adopted to streamline data management, enhance access to records by patients, and improve communication among various healthcare service providers.
- Telemedicine and Remote Care: With increased development in telecommunication technologies, one can have virtual consultations, monitor from a distance, and even provide telehealth services, thereby increasing access to care with lessened geographical barriers.
- IoT and Wearable Devices: Wearable health gadgets pop up, and technology enables ubiquitous health monitoring through IoT to enable early detection of health problems and personalized health management.
- AI and Machine Learning: AI and machine learning algorithms in diagnostics, predictive analytics for decision-making, and personalized treatment recommendations—the convincing prowess of decision-making and operational efficiencies is overwhelming.

2.2.1.2 Policy Reforms and Regulatory Changes

- Healthcare Reform Initiatives: There are government policies and healthcare reforms, such as the Affordable Care Act in the United States of America, initiated to bring about improvement in accessibility to healthcare, reduction of costs, and enhancement in the quality of care.
- Data Privacy Regulations: Laws such as the Health Insurance Portability and Accountability Act and the General Data Protection Regulation have set standards for data privacy and security, further increasing trust and compliance in the practice of digital health.

2.2.1.3 Shifting Patient Expectations

- Engaged Patient Empowerment: The patient of today, while enlightened about health matters through digital platforms, hungers even more for personalized and participatory care.
- Convenience and Accessibility: The convenience and availability in all these digital health tools and telemedicine services breed the desire to meet patient demands for access to healthcare that better accommodates schedules and lifestyles.

2.2.1.4 Pursuit of Improved Health Outcomes

- Emphasis on Prevention Care: Data analytics and wearable technologies promise a growing emphasis on preventive care and early intervention, enabling proactive management of health and chronic conditions.
- Personalized Medicine: In the advance of genomics and pharmacogenomics, focus would shift to personalized medicine using customized treatment per individual genetic profile and specific health needs with the guarantee of effectiveness and more targeted therapies.

2.2.1.5 Cost Efficiency and Value-Based Care

- Move to Value-Based Care Models: Many health systems are adopting value-based models. The latter are based on patient outcomes and cost-effectiveness, with a challenge of controlling the cost of care amidst improved quality.
- Optimization of Resources: These technological innovations, along with the use of big data, facilitate better use of resources. Overall efficiencies within health improve, with the reduction of waste.

All these factors are driving the current development in the healthcare sector. They enable innovations that help raise the bar regarding care delivery and patient outcome and overall efficiency of the system. These will continue to evolve and, likely, further change and innovate the healthcare landscape (Kasoju et al. 2023).

2.3 Digital Transformation in Health

The digital transformation in health has been the paradigm shift that has completely changed the way medical services were delivered and managed. It is driven by EHRs replacing traditional paper-based systems for better, more accurate management of patient information, improving coordination among healthcare providers, and facilitating real-time access to critical health data. Telemedicine, being in the limelight, was considered to increase access by allowing patients to consult with healthcare professionals remotely and thereby bridge gaps in healthcare delivery, especially in remote and underserved areas. Integration of wearable devices with IoT technology has revolutionized patient care as it can continuously monitor the health metrics of patients, promptly detect potential issues, and manage personalized health by collecting data in real time. mHealth applications have also empowered patients to be more proactive in managing their health, adhering to fitness goals, and easily accessing medical information via smartphones. All in all, these digital advances have paved the way for streamlined processes, active patient participation, and a better-informed and more accessible healthcare system to prove that a sea change has taken place in how healthcare services are envisioned and delivered in the modern era (Lerzynski 2021).

2.3.1 *Adoption of EHRs*

Electronic healthcare records (EHR) adoption is a paradigm-shifting phenomenon in the care sector, changing the way information about the patient is recorded, accessed, and utilized. Replacing traditional paper-based medical records, EHRs introduced digitized systems that boast a variety of advantages in handling patient data. EHR centralizes and digitizes patient information, improving the comprehensiveness and accuracy of the medical record, reducing manual record-keeping errors, and enhancing quality of care. It lets providers access the complete history of the patient: previous diagnoses, plans of treatment, and results of tests from one source for better decisions and coordination of care provided by multiple providers in multiple settings.

EHR integration also smoothed the administrative process by handling appointments, billing, and documentation, hence increasing efficiency and reducing operations costs. Other functions provided in many of the EHR systems include electronic prescribing, which improves medication safety due to decreased prescription errors and real-time drug interaction checks. EHRs also enable great communication between healthcare professionals and patients through secure messaging and patient portals that afford the individual the opportunity to access his or her health record, monitor his or her progress, and actively participate in his or her care.

Further still, EHRs provide the critical mechanism for collecting and analyzing data that informs public health research and epidemiological studies via large-scale datasets. It also allows the development of health trends, evaluation of results of treatment, and the implementation of evidence-based practices. Moreover, there are some barriers to EHR adoption, including high initial investment, maintenance costs, data privacy, and security issues. Despite such challenges, the benefits that EHRs can achieve—improved accuracy, efficiency, and greater patient involvement—signal it is well-placed to play a critical role in fostering an integrated, data-driven health sector.

2.3.2 *Growth of Telemedicine*

Growth in telemedicine signifies that the future of healthcare has been revolutionized, for it has changed the way consultations and treatment are pursued. In other words, telemedicine is the mode of accessing health services through digital technologies related to communication remotely. Certainly, it widened access to healthcare by bypassing geographical constraints and bringing convenience to patients.

Such development has been supported by technology innovations such as videoconferencing, mobile health apps, and secure messaging, allowing simultaneous activity exchange between the patients and their health professionals. However, telemedicine has been most transformative in areas that are either underserved or rural, where access to health facilities and specialists is very poor. Telemedicine allows remote consultations, bridging discontinuations in the delivery of healthcare; patients receive medical advice, diagnosis, and treatment plans without necessarily having to make long journeys to facilities. It has improved access to care, reduced waiting times, and enhanced the efficiency of healthcare delivery.

The COVID-19 pandemic accelerated the adoption of telemedicine rapidly, as social distancing and lockdowns created an imperative for remote healthcare solutions. In such a setting, it proved invaluable for continuity of care, management of chronic conditions, and mental health support while minimizing virus transmission. The pandemic also provided temporary changes in some regulatory requirements and expanded insurance coverages for services delivered via telemedicine, further contributing to its sustained growth and increased acceptance. Other advantages of telemedicine include increased access and convenience but also a potential reduction in costs associated with in-person visits through reductions in transportation expenses, as well as overhead costs associated with maintaining physical healthcare facilities. Other benefits of telemedicine are continuous monitoring and follow-up of patients, which are very relevant to the management of chronic conditions and prevention.

Despite the advantages, disadvantages in telemedicine include concerns about the fair access of the concerned technology, data privacy, and security, and integration into conventional healthcare systems. Despite this fact, continuous development regarding telemedicine technologies and awareness of their benefits foresees that this modality will remain an important driver in the healthcare scenario, always seeking further innovation and improvement of healthcare delivery over these years (Takahashi et al. 2022).

2.3.3 Impact of Wearable Devices and IoT

The wearable devices coupled with the Internet of Things (IoT) has altered healthcare to the level where it is possible to manage health in a proactive manner and care for patients on personal levels. Examples of wearable devices are fitness trackers, smartwatches, and health monitors in real time, using various biometric data on your body—for example, heart rate variability, activity, sleep, and glucose levels. Such metrics, tracked on a continual basis, allow one to get insights into their health status and to set personal health goals about such metrics—further monitoring their progress toward achieving the set goals.

Finally, health can even be greatly improved with the integration of IoT technology into healthcare. That is made possible by allowing wearable devices to connect to a network with other smart health devices and systems. Health data can be shared wirelessly through IoT sensors to the care provider, which allows remote health monitoring and early-stage presence detection. For instance, IoT-connected glucose monitors can send alerts on potential blood sugar level anomalies both to patients and health professionals for timely management of diabetes. In addition, smart home devices like connected weighing scales and blood pressure monitors support holistic health tracking and management. This impact of wearable devices and IoT goes further to include preventive care and early detection of health issues. Continuous monitoring identifies patterns and anomalies in data that might suggest the emergence of a medical condition, allowing for early intervention that reduces the risk of serious health events. The proactive approach in health management not only brings about improved outcomes at an individual level but also contributes to the public health through valued data provision for research and disease surveillance. Wearable devices and IoT enhance the engagement of patients in health and adherence to follow-up. All these technologies have positive impacts because they facilitate real-time feedback and personalized health information, which, in turn, may motivate patients for self-management and compliance about lifestyle improvement or medication intake. This will result in better patient outcomes and more effective use of health resources.

With such pervasive adoption of wearables and IoT in healthcare, those challenges like data privacy, security, and interoperability issues seem very nearly bound to occur. Data privacy and security issues are paramount, and integration of data from different devices into single health records in a coherent manner seems to be another key issue required for the successful unwinding of such technologies. These are not without the many challenges that wearable devices, along with IoT, face; this really reflects huge implications for the future of healthcare in relation to health monitoring, early detection of potential problems in health, and improved patient engagement.

2.3.4 Mobile Health (mHealth) Applications

Mobile health applications represent the next level of revolution in healthcare, using the ubiquity created by smartphones and other mobile devices to create in the delivery of health-related services and information directly to the consumer. These range from monitoring health to symptom checkers, managing medications, and even telemedicine consultations, while resources on maintaining wellness increase accessibility and personalization.

mHealth applications enable continuous health monitoring by tracking health metrics in physical activities, dietary behaviors, sleeping patterns, and vital signs. Most of these applications are endowed with goal setting for health parameters, personalized recommendations, and time-related trend analysis to ensure that individuals act regarding their health and well-being. Such as the fact that fitness and activity trackers can show results in mHealth applications, which can return immediate feedback related to exercising routines, guides nutrition and meal planning through dietary apps.

The other area where the influence of mHealth applications is very important is in medical management. The adherence apps may also remind the patients about their medication schedule, inform them about drug interactions, and track their intake while guiding and supporting the patients for compliance with the prescribed drug regimen and reducing the chances of a missed dose or any other type of medication error.

Complementary to these is the trend of telemedicine, complemented by mHealth applications designed to allow for virtual consultations between patients and healthcare providers. Such applications include video calling, secure messaging, and appointment settings, which make it easier for patients to access medical services without necessarily physically visiting a healthcare facility. This has been among other things instrumental in managing chronic conditions, specialist advice, as well as non-emergency health problems.

Other mHealth applications provide support for mental health and wellness by offering resources on stress management, mindfulness, and emotional support. For example, mental health applications provide tools to understand cognitive-behavioral therapy, mood tracking, and relaxation exercises, which in turn allow self-management of overall mental well-being and disease states such as anxiety and depression.

While mHealth applications can provide accessibility, convenience, and personalization among other pros, applications are generally faced with a host of challenges with regard to data privacy and security and quality of information. Ensuring security of personal health data and verification for accuracy will be paramount in gaining user trust and effectiveness. However, this growth and development of mHealth applications do suggest that they hold enormous potential both to enhance healthcare delivery while at the same time empowering individuals in maintaining their health and improving health outcomes (Gagneja and Gagneja 2015).

2.4 Personalized Medicine

Personalized medicine is a revolutionary vision for healthcare because it allows treatment to be tailored to the unique qualities of everyone: their genome, lifestyle, and environment. That is where medicine moves away from the one-size-fits-all model, embracing genomics, data analytics, and precision medicine for more targeted therapies. Through genetic makeup, health professionals may now pinpoint very specific biomarkers and genetic mutations linked with diseases, therefore developing targeted treatments which deal with the root cause of the disease rather than the symptoms. It improves the efficacy of the treatment while minimizing adverse drug responses, hence making the processes of early detection and prevention by predictive tests possible. It also interlaces data from analytics and artificial intelligence to develop treatment strategies for better patient outcomes. Thus, personalized medicine makes for a more personalized, proactive, patient-centered healthcare with great promise in managing chronic diseases, preventing diseases, and ensuring better health.

2.4.1 Advances in Genomics and Precision Medicine

Genomics and precision medicine are revolutionary due to the change in approach towards personalized medical treatment based on an individual's peculiar characteristics. Moreover, such advances have greatly increased our understanding of genetic influences on health and disease, leading to treatments that are targeted and effective.

Genomics is the study of a person's entire genome; hence, all his genes interact with one another and with the environment. Sequencing of the human genome thanks to the Human Genome Project mapped out human genetic information and enabled further investigations into predispositions and mechanisms of diseases at a genetic level. This basic knowledge accelerated genomic technologies like NGS, which allows for the swift and affordable analysis of genetic information. These technologies have empowered the researcher and the clinician with the facility to define variants in genes that are associated with diseases: cancer, cardiovascular conditions, and rare genetic disorders (Quazi 2022).

Precision medicine utilizes genomic advances by applying such genetic knowledge to tailored healthcare strategies, each suited to an individual patient. While old methods apply a one-size-fits-all treatment approach, precision medicine accordingly elaborates intervention based on an individual's genetic background plus his or her life and environmental concerns. By personalizing treatment, this increases efficacy while lessening the chances of adverse effects. In oncology, for example, genomic profiling of tumors can identify specific genetic mutations driving tumor growth, where targeted therapies destroy cancerous cells with such mutations, sparing healthy cells in the process.

Pharmacogenomics is the subclass of precision medicine that involves how genetic variability within an individual can affect response to medication. Pharmacogenomics analyzes genetic factors which affect drug metabolism and effectiveness, thereby enabling treatment by healthcare providers through the prescription of medications that are most likely to be effective but with minimal side effects for each patient. This not only enhances treatment outcomes but also reduces the trial-and-error process often associated with finding the right medication.

The place of genomics and precision medicine within the clinical realm has been further supported by the development of genomic databases and their constituent bioinformatics tools that will enable the interpretation and application of genetic information. Such collaborations by researchers, clinicians, and data scientists will finally allow the translation of genomic information into everyday healthcare to bring us closer to personalized treatment plans and preventive approaches.

While both genomics and precision medicine hold promise, challenges persist, such as data-privacy issues, ethical considerations, and the need for comprehensive genetic counseling. Ensuring equitable access to these advanced technologies is of importance, along with the response to potential disparities in genetic testing and treatment. With research at an ever-evolving pace and technology constantly improving, genomics and precision medicine are in a very good position to alter healthcare by offering increasingly tailored, effective, and proactive approaches to the prevention and treatment of disease.

2.4.2 Development of Tailored Treatments and Therapies

Genomics and precision medicine represent the leading edge in a new changing medical paradigm that will increasingly focus on tailoring medical treatment to unique features of each individual patient. Such developments have greatly advanced our knowledge of genetic influences on health and disease, hence contributing to the availability of less generalized and more specific therapies.

Genomics is, therefore, the study of all genes that exist within an individual, how they interact with one another, and how they interact with the environment. The sequencing of the human genome—through efforts like the Human Genome Project—has presented a map of human genetic information, after which time deeper insight into genetic predispositions and mechanisms of disease have been found possible. This basic knowledge acted as the catalyst for further progress in genomic technologies, including NGS, which can rapidly analyze genetic data at much lower costs. These technologies will enable researchers and clinicians to identify the genetic variants underlying many human conditions, such as cancer, cardiovascular diseases, and rare genetic disorders.

Precision medicine uses this advancement in genomics by taking this genetic knowledge to translate into the tailoring of health strategies according to the unique conditions and needs of the individual patient. Precision medicine styles interventions based on an individual's genetic profile and lifestyle, along with environmental factors, instead of the generalized treatment model of the traditional approach. This provides a personalized solution that will be highly effective and reduce the aftereffects. For example, in oncology, tumor genomic profiling may hint at genetic mutations driving tumor growth that permit treatments targeted against cancerous cells harboring those mutations and spare healthy tissue.

Pharmacogenomics is a subcategory of precision medicine that explains how the variability in the genetic information of a particular individual gives rise to a differential response to medicines. Pharmacogenomics will enable health practitioners to prescribe medications with increased effectiveness and safety for any given patient, through the assessment of genetic factors deciding upon drug metabolism and efficacy. This approach improves the treatment outcome and diminishes the hit-and-miss process that was earlier experienced in finding the right medication.

This has been further supported by the creation of large-scale genomic databases and bioinformatics tools that permit the interpretation and application of genetic data. Such items and the help provided through cooperative efforts of the researchers, clinicians, and data scientists lead to constant advancement in the ability to integrate genomic information into actual healthcare, with the final goal of personalizing treatments and preventive strategies.

At the same time, challenges highlighted refer to those that relate to data privacy and sensitive ethical issues, coupled with the insufficiency of expertly given comprehensive genetic counseling. This way, it is ensured that benefits of all these new and sophisticated technologies are genuinely availed with equal opportunities and solutions to avert potential disparities in genetic testing and treatment. Since research and technology continue to be advanced even today, abundant opportunities for further development lie ahead in genomics and precision medicine. These will help transform healthcare in realizing more effective, efficient, and timely ways of disease prevention and treatment, with a patient-centered approach.

Personalized treatment and therapy have been one of the major milestones in modern medicine, stemming from the integration of genomics, precision medicine, and state-of-the-art analytics. This approach makes every effort to tailor medical treatment to the specific genetic, environmental, and lifestyle factors of the individual to enhance the potential of treatment and reduce the risk of adverse events.

Targeted treatments are informed by the knowledge that genetic variability in people determines how they may respond to certain drugs and therapies. By analyzing the genetic makeup of a patient, health professionals can ascertain the exact biomarkers or genetic mutations for any given condition. Such information can then be used to develop targeted therapies aimed at addressing the very causes of the disease and not its symptoms. In this regard, targeted treatments, interfering in certain molecular pathways related to carcinogenesis, for example, in oncology, are more effective and less toxic than classical chemotherapy.

Pharmacogenomics is one of the pivotal parts of tailored therapy development that deals with the capability to assess how genetic variability changes drug metabolism and the effectiveness of such drugs. It aids in identifying potential adverse or inadequate responses to specific medications, which, in turn, enables the health practitioner to adjust the drug choice or dose. As an example, this may help when prescribing anticoagulants like warfarin, guiding the optimal dosage based on genetic testing for variants that affect drug metabolism and hence avoid a bleeding risk (Jain 2021).

Furthermore, biomarker discovery plays a very important role in the realization of personalized therapies. Biomarkers are measurable indicators of biological processes or responses to treatment; their identification may help direct an optimal therapeutic approach—for example, in an oncology scenario where the identification of specific tumor markers will help the oncologist decide on the most effective chemotherapy regimen or whether the patient should receive targeted biological agents.

These have progressively taken on a current approach toward the use of advanced data analytics and machine learning to analyze complex datasets from genomics, clinical records, and patient outcomes. Technologies enable the uncovering of patterns and associations that preserve the development of customized therapies. Predictive models can make predictions about how patients are likely to respond to various treatments in efforts to enhance optimized therapy plans and accelerate decision-making.

Clinical trials nowadays are being designed in approaches of personalized medicine, often considering the actual design for specific genetic or molecular subgroups of patients. This stratified approach allows the more precise assessment of efficacy and safety within the population targeted, leading to more reliable and clinically relevant results.

Despite the promise of therapies and treatments tailored to the individual, challenges include ensuring there is robust evidence to support their effectiveness, issues related to cost and accessibility, and integrating personalized approaches into routine clinical practice. Thus, this depends on various serious challenges that must be overcome if the full impact of tailored treatments in improving patient outcomes and advancing medicine as a field is ever going to be realized through further research and technology.

2.4.3 Impact of Personalized Medicine on Patient Outcomes

Personalized medicine has revolutionized patient outcomes by giving specialized medical care to unique genetics, environmental, and lifestyle modalities. That allows for more specific treatment and better efficacy, hence enhancing health outcomes and providing a more personalized model of healthcare for the patients.

Better Therapeutic Effect: The very essence of personalized medicine involves healthcare providers deciding on treatment, taking into consideration a person's genetic profile and particular characteristics of his or her disease. For example, tumor genomic profiling in oncology may disclose specific mutations responsible for the growth of a tumor and thus allow the use of targeted therapies that are more effective against such mutations. It is such precision that decreases ineffective treatments and increases better therapeutic outcomes.

Fewer Side Adverse Effects: Medication specifically based on the person's genetics minimizes harmful side effects and drug reactions. It therefore permits a pharmacogenomics—considered an improvement in the optimum dosing of medicines and selection, which reduces injurious side effects and improves safety and overall tolerability of a treatment.

Better Disease Management: With personalized medicine, the condition of the patient and its progression are better understood. In cases of a chronic disease, such as diabetes or cardiovascular conditions, personalized treatment plans that consider genetic predispositions along with lifestyle factors can help in the more effective management and control of the disease for better long-term outcomes.

Principle of Early Detection and Prevention: Personalized medicine also goes out to extend its use in early detection and preventive care. Genetic screening and risk assessments identify individuals who are at high risk for certain diseases while asymptomatic, therefore prompting early intervention and preventive care. For example, genetic testing may determine the genetic predisposition to diseases like breast cancer or cardiovascular disease, thereby allowing the implementation of early monitoring and prevention strategies that could reduce disease incidence and improve prognosis.

Optimized Drug Development: Since personalized medicine fits better with certain genetic or molecular profiles, it further affects patient outcomes in new therapies development. Accordingly, clinical trials can be designed to consider personalized approaches, which may pinpoint subgroups of patients most likely to benefit from new treatments, hence developing more efficient and effective processes for drug development.

Personalized medicine increases patient engagement through care decision-making and treatment planning. Secondly, when treatments address unique patient characteristics, there is usually higher satisfaction and adherence from patients to the prescribed regime. This type of activity in care can promote a better relationship between the patient and provider, further leading to improved health outcomes in general.

While personalized medicine does boast several benefits, some of the challenges include very extensive genetic testing, issues over the privacy of data, and equitable access to personalized treatment. Meeting these challenges will be important in maximizing positive impact on patient outcomes and in moving the science further toward a more personalized and effective healthcare system (Ghebrehiwet et al. 2024).

2.5 Data Analytics and Artificial Intelligence (AI)

Data analytics and AI are improving care fundamentally by the way data improves patient outcomes, streamlines operations, and advances medical research. Each technology offers powerful tools to analyze vast amounts of health data, develop actionable insights, and optimize healthcare delivery.

Data Analytics: The process consists of a detailed analysis of complex health data to find patterns, trends, and correlations that may inform clinical decisions and operational improvements. It therefore helps to interpret the data emanating from EHRs, wearable devices, and other digital channels, at increased volumes, toward better results in patient outcomes. For example, predictive analytics uses historical data with statistical algorithms to forecast probable health events in the future, such as the likelihood of hospital readmission or risk of chronic diseases. This proactive strategy by the providers helps in the instigation of prevention and customized therapy plans, hence improving the management of the patients.

Artificial Intelligence: This involves various technologies, including machine learning, natural language processing, and deep learning, which all can undertake tasks generally performed by the human cognitive mechanism to analyze and interpret complex data. Applications of AI in healthcare include the following:

The AI algorithms for diagnostic assistance may use medical images such as X-rays, MRI, and CT. This helps the radiologist in higher accuracy during diagnosis. Image analysis can help in the early detection of diseases like cancers, using AI-powered tools with much greater precision than conventional methods.

Personalized Treatment Plans: With the integrated data, such as genetic information and patient health records, AI models can provide customized treatment plans. Considering the characteristics a patient possesses along with a predictive response for various therapies, AI treats them more personally and effectively.

Predictive Analytics: AI uses predictive modeling to forecast needs and outcomes in patients. For instance, it can predict the complications that might be witnessed in patients, depicted from their health data, to allow for early interventions and management strategies that are targeted.

The algorithms of NLP would cruise through unstructured data from the clinical notes and other textual sources, which may be seen as valuable information. It enhances the integration of information to strengthen clinical research while promoting evidence-based decision-making on different broad-level data sources.

Operational Efficiency: AI-driven innovations optimize the administrative process, including scheduling, billing, and resource planning. Automated systems can create automated workflows to reduce their administrative burden and further improve efficiency in healthcare.

With data analytics coupled with AI, diagnosis accuracy will be higher, treatment options will be more personalized, and operational efficiency in healthcare will improve. However, there are challenges yet to be overcome, such as data privacy, the need for high-quality data, and ethical issues with AI decision-making. Ensuring that responsibilities and equity in the use of such technologies are duly considered will better position such technologies to achieve maximum potential in improving quality of care. As these technologies continue to evolve, no doubt data analytics and AI will move to center stage in shaping healthcare's future (Murphy and Feeney 2023).

2.5.1 Role of Big Data in Healthcare

Big data has surged to the forefront as one of healthcare's most critical factors, enabling enormous volumes and an array of data types to unleash analytics, patient outcomes, and system efficiencies. These include not only EHRs and medical imaging but also genetic data, wearables, and patient surveys, among others. These data give a fuller view into an individual and population health.

Enhanced Patient Care: Big data can offer a complete vision of patient health by integrating data from various sources. This enables very accurate diagnoses and the design of personalized treatment plans. For example, data from EHRs and wearable devices can be analyzed for patterns and trends in order to predict health issues well in advance so that timely interventions may be made with appropriate care strategies.

Predictive Analytics and Risk Management: Big data analytics can predict future health risks and outcomes through identification of trends and patterns in large datasets. Using predictive models allows for the determination of risk regarding diseases, hospital readmissions, and responses to treatments, thus providing opportunities for healthcare professionals to establish preventive measures and personalize treatments. This proactive approach leads to better patient management and reduces the incidence of preventable conditions.

Operational Efficiency: Big data smoothens the operations of healthcare by optimizing resource utilization, reducing administrative costs, and increasing workflow efficiency. Data-driven insight can improve scheduling, reduce wait times, and underpin better decision-making in resource management. Analyzing patient flow data can also help hospitals manage bed occupancy better and allocate staff accordingly.

Population Health Management: Big data provides analytics related to health trends in the population, which is the basis for developing public health initiatives and policy decisions. Based on data from a variety of sources, health organizations identify health disparities and track outbreaks of diseases. It also estimates the outcomes and impacts of major public health programs. Targeted interventions and strategies to improve outcomes regarding community health are based on this information.

Research and Development: The movement of large amounts of data accelerates medical research; it provides researchers with datasets through which they can test new treatments, identify biomarkers, and understand the mechanism of a disease. Big data works by analyzing clinical trial results, genomic information, and real-world evidence to drive innovation in the development of drugs and treatments.

Big data also enables patient engagement by creating avenues for patients' access to their personal health information and insights through patient portals and mobile applications. The transparency accorded to them will enable the patients to track their health metrics, understand their conditions, and make informed decisions about their care.

While big data in health projects several benefits, there are challenges associated with it, relating to data privacy and security, interoperability of systems, and ethics around the use of data. These will have to be tackled if the full benefit of big data is to be harnessed toward better healthcare provision and patient outcomes. Big data in healthcare will continue to shape the future of medicine through advancements in personalized care, operational efficiency, and public health as technology continues to evolve.

2.5.2 Applications of AI and Machine Learning in Diagnostics

Artificial intelligence and machine learning are revolutionizing the diagnostics field with their sophisticated algorithms and models in an effort to increase the capability, efficiency, and speed in disease detection and diagnosis. Technology uses volumes of data to identify patterns, make predictions, and support healthcare professionals in making better decisions.

Medical Imaging Analysis: AI and ML algorithms have been phenomenally successful in analyzing medical images, including X-rays, MRI, and CT scans. Training on large datasets of labeled images helps algorithms spot abnormalities like tumors, fractures, and lesions with accuracy. For instance, AI systems can detect early signs of cancer, such as breast and lung cancer, from mammograms or chest X-rays, respectively, with a high level of diagnostic accuracy compared to human radiologists, minimizing the possibility of missed diagnosis.

AI and ML in pathology have been employed to examine tissue samples for biopsy results. Machine learning models interpret complex histopathological images, detecting the presence of cancerous cells, classify tumor types, and determine disease progression. Automation of this process will not only speed up the time taken for diagnosis but also improve consistency and reliability in reports from pathology.

Genomic Diagnostics: AI and ML are integral in genomic data analysis to help in the identification of genetic mutations and variations that predispose individuals to a number of diseases. These technologies interpret large-scale genomic sequences, identify biomarkers, and predict disease risk using genetic profiles. For instance, AI might be used to diagnose rare genetic disorders by comparing patient genomes to large reference databases for potentially pathogenic variant identification.

Predictive Analytics: The machine learning models predict the possibility of certain conditions from data provided by the patient, such as EHR, lifestyle factors, and genetics. Predictive analytics may foresee disease risk, including those disorders pertaining to cardiovascular events or diabetes, for which early intervention and precautionary measures may be very necessary. These models thereby enable providers of healthcare to identify high-risk patients and tailor appropriate screening and monitoring strategies.

CDSS: Clinical decision support systems, nurtured by AI, provide diagnostic suggestions to healthcare professionals in real time, based on patient data. These integrate various data, including medical history, laboratory test results, and imaging studies that provide evidence-based suggestions and support clinical decisions. The CDSS has the potential to point out possible diagnoses, propose proper tests, and indicate choices of therapy that will enable the enhancement of diagnostic precision and quality of patient care.

Natural Language Processing: Techniques in NLP enable information to be extracted from unstructured data such as clinical notes and medical records. AI models can read and classify this text data into diagnosing conditions based on documented symptoms, patient history, and physician notes. NLP enhances the capabilities of diagnostic data extraction and enables comprehensive patient assessment.

Real-Time Monitoring: AI and ML find their applications in real-time monitoring systems that are continuously utilized in the assessment of patient health data from wearables and remote sensors. Examples include the early detection of warning signs in medical conditions such as arrhythmias or sepsis to alert healthcare providers for timely and proper intervention. Real-time analytics offer dynamic and responsive diagnostic approaches that improve patient outcomes and increase care efficiency.

While AI and machine learning hold much promise for diagnostics, data quality, algorithm transparency, and integration with existing healthcare systems are just some of the challenges that have to be resolved. Ensuring the ethical use of AI while taking a complementary approach between technology and health professionals is vital to derive full benefits from these innovations for diagnostic practices (Milan 2023).

2.5.3 Predictive Analytics and Proactive Healthcare

Predictive analytics are making a shift in proactive healthcare by integrating data with sophisticated algorithms that project health trends and determine risks for early intervention. On the contrary, it shifts the paradigm from being reactive to proactive; this would, in fact, enable caregivers to predict any possible health problem well in advance and implement strategies to prevent the same.

Predictive analytics leveraging multiple sources of data historical and real time—from EHRs, wearable sensors, and genetic sources are integral to risk assessment and early detection. For example, predictive models mine patient data to predict the possibility of the onset of chronic diseases like diabetes, cardiovascular disease, or cancer. Identifying persons at higher risk can enable healthcare providers to recommend lifestyle changes, preventive screenings, and early interventions that may prevent or minimize risk factors and ensure optimal long-term health outcomes.

Personalized Health Management: Predictive analytics enables personalized health management through the development of specific prevention and treatment plans considering the risk profile. Classic algorithms analyze genetic, environmental, and lifestyle variables for personalized recommendations on nutrition, exercise, and medication. This approach increases not only the effectiveness of interventions but also active patient involvement in, and compliance with, health recommendations.

Resource planning can be smoothened and optimized by predictive analytics in health systems through predictions of need and demand for patients. For instance, predictive models may project admission rates, volume of emergency room visits, or bed occupancy rates. This therefore enables the health facilities to make better preparations and management decisions related to resources, optimizes wait times, and enhances service provision. This is a proactive approach whereby health organizations may estimate surges or dips in the volume of patients that are coming in for better operations.

Chronic Disease Management: Predictive analytics plays a very important role in managing chronic diseases through monitoring patient data to bring out early signs of worsening conditions. For example, predictive models developed for the management of diabetes will consider glucose levels, activity data, and medication adherence to forecast further complications that might arise or episodes of hypoglycemia. This will provide timely adjustments in treatment plans and preventive measures that avoid serious health events.

Population Health Management: On a larger scale, predictive analytics enables the management of population health through the analysis of trends and patterns across large populations. It is data-driven in nature, enhancing the identification of public health issues, the tracking of disease outbreaks, and the assessment of the effectiveness of health interventions. For example, predictive models can monitor the trends of a flu season and predict outbreaks, hence allowing public health authorities to better position resources and vaccination campaigns.

Clinical Decision Support: Predictive analytics amplify clinical decision-making through data-driven insights and recommendations provided to healthcare professionals. The decision support systems embed the predictive models with patient information in order to provide real-time support about diagnosis, treatment options, and care plans. This sort of support assists clinicians in arriving at informed decisions, improving diagnostic precision, and choosing the most suitable interventions for individual patients.

Patient Engagement and Self-Management: Predictive analytics provides the power of insight into health risks and progress, thus enabling patients to take a very active interest in their health. Through mobile apps and patient portals, individuals will have access to predictive information on their health status, receive personalized recommendations, and track their progress toward health goals. This process of engagement will accelerate a proactive attitude toward health, thus promoting adherence to preventive measures and treatment plans.

Predictive analytics can make a significant contribution to proactive healthcare. The issues that remain to be resolved are by no means least those relating to data privacy, the accuracy of algorithms, and the integration with existing systems. Ethical use of predictive analytics and retaining patient trust must be fostered and looked after if greater use is to be derived from these technologies in reinforcing preventative care and improving outcomes.

2.5.4 AI in Drug Discovery and Development

Artificial intelligence will revolutionize both drug discovery and development by accelerating the identification of new therapies, optimally designing drugs, and improving efficiency in clinical trials. AI technologies, including machine learning, deep learning, and natural language processing, provide effective means to analyze sophisticated biological data, predict drug interactions, and improve the overall drug development pipeline.

Target Identification and Validation: Large-scale genomic, proteomic, and transcriptomic data are analyzed using various AI algorithms to identify and validate new potential targets of drugs. The interactions between genes, proteins, and diseases can be found by machine learning models in order to locate a new target for drug design. For example, AI can process data from high-throughput screening experiments and indicate those proteins or pathway systems that are playing a vital role in the progress of diseases that would direct the research towards new therapeutic targets.

AI with machine learning will facilitate designing and optimizing drug candidates, including the prediction of how a compound will interact with a biological target. AI may utilize computational models to analyze the chemical structure for prediction of binding affinities, and optimization of molecular properties can be performed in order to enhance drug efficacy and reduce potential side effects. Deep learning-based algorithms, as generative models, are also able to design new molecules with the desired properties, thus accelerating the discovery of promising drug candidates.

Predictive Modeling and Simulation: AI-driven predictive modeling and simulation capabilities enable researchers to foresee the actions of drugs in biological systems. Such models simulate interactions of drugs, their metabolism, and pharmacokinetics that provide valuable insights into drug safety and efficacy long before clinical trials. AI can help mitigate the risks of failures at later stages by predictions about potential adverse reactions and optimization of dosing regimens.

Biomarker Identification: AI speeds up the process of biomarker identification that could be used for disease diagnosis, prognosis, and treatment response monitoring. By analyzing large-scale datasets from clinical trials and patient samples, AI can pinpoint patterns and correlations that might indicate biomarkers. These will help develop more precise and personalized therapies and also in the identification of subgroups of patients who might derive the most benefit from certain treatments.

AI enhances the design and recruitment of clinical trials by analyzing patient data to predictively identify those patients who will be suitable candidates for treatment. Machine learning algorithms can consider the genetic profiles of a patient, medical history, and characteristics of a disease in order to match patients with those trials that offer them the best chance of success. In this way, it can reduce recruitment times and increase success rates. The optimization of trial design by

AI involves the forecasting of potential problems, and protocols are adjusted to help in enhancing trial efficiency, which increases the rate of success.

Integration and Analysis: AI is particularly adept at integrating a wide range of data from a number of different sources, including electronic health records, genomic data, and the results of clinical trials. Advanced analytics platforms unleash AI, providing the only holistic view of R&D processes needed to benchmark trends and extract actionable insights from such data. This integrated approach bolsters decision-making and supports a far more efficient drug development pipeline.

AI continues beyond approval to monitor the safety and effectiveness of a drug in its real-world condition. The algorithms will analyze electronic health records, social media, and patient reports to identify adverse events, patterns defining these events, and long-term drug outcomes. In such a direction, continuous monitoring assures the safety of drugs and makes it a basis for their future improvement.

However, not all transformative AI's possibilities in drug discovery and development can be availed without addressing challenges related to data quality, algorithmic transparency, and regulatory consideration. Therefore, it is imperative that standards related to the robustness and reliability of these models are established and further maintained for ethical standards for their application to move the field at a better level overall in drug development. As these AI technologies continue to evolve, they promise to make the process of drug discovery even faster, more accurate, and successful.

2.5.5 *Patient-Centered Care and Empowerment*

Patient-centered care is a paradigm shift in health in which all the needs, preferences, and values of the patients concerning their care are kept first. It means treating individuals as active partners in their health management through the promotion of autonomy for them, ensuring that decisions about their care are made in concordance with the individuals' goals and values. In this view, empowerment is then defined as a process used to equip persons with the necessary knowledge, skills, and support that would enable them to make informed decisions regarding their health status and participate in their care more positively.

Patient-centered care requires every medical treatment and health-keeping strategy to be tailored in close collaboration with the patient, taking into consideration his or her specific needs and personal preferences. This personalization of care can only be addressed through an in-depth understanding of the history of the patient regarding disease and health conditions, his or her lifestyle, and personal objectives. Such influences can help professionals devise treatment plans more relevant and hence effective for each of their patients, thereby enhancing the overall experience and satisfaction with care.

At the heart of patient-centered care lies shared decision-making, a process whereby healthcare providers and patients come together to make informed choices about treatment options. It involves the transmission of full information regarding condition, treatment options, and probable outcomes, encouraging the voicing of patients' preferences and concerns. Shared decision-making keeps a partnership relation of patients and healthcare providers where preferences can be more reflective of the patient's values and better adherence to treatment.

Patient Education and Engagement: Empowerment through education is a very critical component of patient-centered care. Through education, in cases where information is relayed to the patients about the state of their health conditions, treatment alternatives, and management, the patient is able to appreciate their role in their care and make sound decisions. Some educational resources that might be suggested include brochures, online tools for health promotion counseling, and patient portals. Mostly, these aim to provide appropriate information coursed out to support the needs of managing one's own health.

Access to Health Information: For healthcare to actually be patient-centered, health information provision should be there for the patient, such as medical records, test results, and treatment plans, among others. Digital tools that assist in viewing health data include patient portals and mobile health applications for monitoring progress and communicating with healthcare providers. In this regard, the transparency built into such an approach develops trust and further empowers patients toward active involvement in care.

Self-Management Support: Empowerment of the patient in engaging and equipping them with the tools is necessary toward successful self-management of their health. This would include access to self-monitoring devices like blood glucose monitors or wearable fitness trackers and instructions on how to effectively use them in managing chronic conditions or tracking health metrics. Coaching, counseling, and peer support groups are such supportive resources that offer equal support towards taking good care of one's health and meeting wellness goals.

Respect for Patient Preferences and Values: The philosophy of patient-centered care demands that healthcare providers respect and integrate the preferences and values of patients into care decisions. It means taking into consideration cultural, religious, and personal convictions that may assist patients in making choices and respecting the desires of the patients with regard to treatment options, care settings, and end-of-life care. In honor of these preferences, healthcare providers will be assured that the care provided is valorized with the patients' values and their overall satisfaction with the healthcare experience.

Improved Outcomes and Satisfaction: Evidence exists that a patient-centered approach tends to lead to better health outcomes, more satisfied patients, and better observance of treatment plans. If patients feel that they are in some control in their care and that their preferences are considered, they are much more likely to adopt healthier behaviors, adhere to treatments, and achieve positive health outcomes. This leads to a more pleasant experience within healthcare, reducing anxiety and therefore increasing the patient's trust in their provider.

It also brings many challenges with its implementation, in the form of equity of access to resources, communication problems, and integration into existing health systems. Solving these, and creating a culture where collaboration and respect form the keystones, will go a long way toward enhancing the perspective on patient-centered care and empowerment to ensure better quality overall and, importantly, improved patient outcomes.

2.6 Emerging Trends and Technologies

Hence, emerging technologies and trends in healthcare are further remodeling with innovative solutions aimed at diagnosis, treatment, and management. Artificial intelligence and machine learning, on one hand, bring a revolution in diagnosis and personalized treatment by decoding big volumes of data into the forecast of patient outcomes and personalized targets of therapy with unparalleled precision. Telemedicine and telehealth have been bridging such access to care, making healthcare even more accessible and convenient. There is immediate feedback that wearable devices and health monitoring technologies are implementing on the vital signs and physical activities of a person, thus empowering proactive health management and early intervention. Advances in genomics drive personalized medicine in targeted treatments with respect to one's genetic profile. Meanwhile, blockchain technology may enhance data security and interoperability. Robotics and automation enhance surgical precision and operational efficiency, while virtual and augmented reality open new ways of carrying out medical education and training. IoMT connects medical devices and systems for real-time health monitoring and efficient coordination of care. 3D printing allows personalization of devices and implants; innovative pharmaceuticals allow for better targeting of drugs. All these together will revolutionize healthcare delivery to become more personalized, efficient, and effective as each of these is continually evolving and integrating into everyday practice.

2.6.1 The Future of Telemedicine and Remote Care

The future in telemedicine and remote care has just reached a juncture where increased access, improved patient outcomes, and efficiency in the care systems are about to materialize. With technology continuing to get better and advanced, it will increasingly play its part in the modern health ecosystem and ease many a problem that may turn out to be quite persistent in traditional in-person care.

Care Expansion: Telemedicine has widened access to health services, especially in areas very far or not served. By allowing video consultations with their healthcare providers, consultations over the phone, or through a secure messaging platform, geographic barriers are reduced, and such patients remain serviced in a timely manner without necessarily having to make a trip for this. This accessibility has particularly made it easy to manage chronic conditions, follow-up cases, and initial consultations.

Integration of Advanced Technologies: Infusing AI and machine learning into telemedicine platforms has been one of the advances in technology, ensuring great accuracy in diagnosis and personalized care. AI-powered tools analyze data and symptoms of patients and suggest outcomes in real time, assist in case triaging, and support decision-making. Beyond this, remote monitoring devices, including wearables and sensors, can monitor health and gather data for proactive, data-driven care around the clock.

More Engaged Patients: The future of telemedicine in patient engagement and self-management is very bright. Digital health tools, such as patient portals and mobile health applications, enable patients to take a more active role in their care by enabling access to their medical record, results of tests, and personalized health insights. This allows for better communication between the patient and the provider, facilitates adherence to a treatment plan, and promotes healthy lifestyle changes.

Improved Care Coordination: Telemedicine promotes better coordination of care through effective communication among providers. Remote care platforms facilitate the sharing of patient information and collaboration among specialists, primary care physicians, and other professionals to afford the best integration in patient care, with less fragmentation in the delivery of healthcare services.

Cost Reduction and Efficiency: Telemedicine can potentially reduce the cost and enhance operational efficiency in healthcare. Limiting in-person visits has the potential to reduce some transport costs, minimize missed appointments, and decrease administrative burdens. Secondly, consultations and monitoring remotely allow workforce streamlining, thus enabling health providers to treat more patients by optimizing resources utilization.

Well-being and Mental Health: Telemedicine is increasingly being considered a tool to meet issues related to mental health and wellness. It brings the therapy, counseling, and psychiatric interventions closer to every household with any form of comfort, discretion, convenience, and choice. Virtual mental health services are convenient and private, which makes it easier for people to seek help while lessening some stigma associated with getting mental health treatment, thus improving access to vital resources in mental health.

Regulatory and Policy Developments: Decisions about the future of telemedicine are going to be made on constantly updated regulatory and policy frameworks. Greater use of telemedicine will create a need for updated regulation and standards that address issues of quality, security, and payment related to remote care services. For sustainable growth in this field, policymakers and healthcare organizations must zero in on issues such as licensure, reimbursement, and data privacy.

Integration with Traditional Models of Care: Telemedicine, over time, is not thought to replace traditional in-person care but is seen as one more mode of care.

Integration of the conventional healthcare model with that of remote care will further offer a hybrid approach, taking into account both the convenience of telemedicine and the benefits of face-to-face interactions where needed. This model ensures comprehensive, flexible care options for patients.

As telemedicine and remote care technologies continue to evolve, they will be central in the shaping of the future of healthcare. By expanding access, improving patient engagement, and more thoroughly coordinating care, their potential should result in a more effective, efficient, and patient-centered delivery of care. Further development and integration of such technologies will fuel the next generation of healthcare delivery—innovations that must be pursued if current challenges are to be met and a more connected, accessible healthcare system developed.

2.6.2 Integrating AI and Robotics in Healthcare

AI and robotics integrated into the health sector remake the entire industry as it enhances precision and improves patient outcomes across key domains of care. The cohabitation of the computational power of AI with the mechanical capabilities of robotics unfolds a synergy that will transform both clinical and operational facets of healthcare for the times to come.

Improved Diagnostic Accuracy: AI algorithms combined with robotic systems improve the accuracy of diagnostics. Applications can be extended to analyzing complex medical data, such as imaging and genetic information, through pattern and anomaly detection that might not be possible with human vision. This, in turn, takes it even further with robotics providing high-precision manipulators to perform or guide diagnostic procedures. Such robotic-assisted image systems enhance the quality of diagnostic scans and the results thereof for early and reliable diagnosis of diseases.

Preciseness During Surgery: This is one of the most salient applications of AI and robotics in the health arena. The robotic systems allow surgeons to perform minimally invasive procedures with increased preciseness and control, as is the case with the da Vinci Surgical System. This is further enhanced by AI through real-time data analytics, predictive analytics, and enhanced visualization techniques. The result of such integration will reduce the risk of complications and decrease the time of recovery and improve surgical outcomes since interventions could now be finer with minimal invasiveness.

Personal Treatment Planning: AI-powered tools are going to be helpful in generating treatment plans and informing on what the patient's probable response to different types of therapies is. Such plans will then be implemented by robotics with utmost preciseness. For instance, AI will take into consideration a patient's genetic background and his or her respective case history and will recommend specific appropriate treatment options for the robotic systems; these will, in turn, indicate exact dosages and techniques to administer those treatments. Their interaction will, therefore, make therapy alignment with the needs of individual patients to ensure maximum effectiveness while minimizing harmful side effects.

Automation of Patient Care: Inpatient care is one of the fields where rapid transformation is taking place due to robotic automation and AI-drive systems. It liberates practitioners to handle more complex care activities, as routine tasks entail delivery of medication, patient monitoring, and hygiene. Continuous monitoring through AI algorithms can detect deviations from normal trends in real time and, just by that fact, warn healthcare providers against impending issues before they worsen. All such integrations enhance patient safety, reduce errors, and improve efficiency for the care extended overall.

Robotic Rehabilitation: These also have a very important role in rehabilitation and physical therapy. Guided AI algorithmic robotic exoskeleton, among other rehabilitation devices, can support patients in the processes necessary for returning strength and mobility after injuries or surgeries. It is a system for targeted therapies, adaptive to individual progress, and personalized rehabilitation experience. AI-driven feedback and adjustment capabilities can assure that therapy will be efficient yet safe, accelerating recovery and improving functional outcomes.

Operational Efficiency: In addition, AI and robotics improve operational efficiency in health facilities. Application of AI algorithms in maximizing scheduling, resource allocation, and workflow management reduces bottlenecks in operations, therefore enhancing efficient delivery of services. Robotics automates administrative tasks such as data entry and inventory management, hence reducing the administrative burden on healthcare staff while minimizing errors. Efficiency is translated into cost savings and improved patient satisfaction.

More Patient Engagement: AI-driven features incorporated into robotic systems include chatbots and virtual assistants, which make it far easier to involve and support the patients. The facilities ensure that at the right time, information is provided or various queries answered, and appointment management and follow-up are facilitated. Robotics and AI do improve communication with patients by providing personalized interaction and speed to meet definite needs of the patients.

Ethical and Practical Issues: Indeed, with the development and implementation of AI and robotics in the health sector comes a lot of benefits. With that also emanates the development of ethical and practical issues such as data privacy, algorithm transparency, and job displacement. Assurance of ethical and effective application of AI and robotic systems requires continuous evaluation, regulation, and collaboration among stakeholders to maintain the trust and safety level in the health sector.

The integration of AI with robotics has the potential to drive huge development not just in the practice of medicine itself but also in the way care is provided and in operational efficiency. Combining the computational power of AI with the precision and versatility of robotics makes healthcare providers able to deliver much more exact, personal, and efficient care, which heralds a new frontier in medical innovation and excellence.

2.7 Conclusion

This, in turn, is rooted in rapid development within digital technologies, personalized medicine, and AI and robotics. All are fundamentally changing the delivery and experience of care across the revolution going on within the health continuum. Expansion of telemedicine and remote care dismantles barriers to access and gives patients convenient and timely health solutions, whereas for service providers it means the possibility to monitor conditions continuously and take action in order to forestall crises associated with chronic conditions. Spurred on by genomics and precision therapies, the rise of personalized medicine tailors treatments to individual genetic profiles for better efficacy and fewer side effects.

Artificial Intelligence and Machine Learning are changing the diagnostic and treatment paradigm through predictive analytics and decision support, raising the quality of care. Robotics improve surgical precision and automate routine tasks in rehabilitation. This results in better patient outcomes and more operational efficiency. Not only are these technologies driving the capabilities of medicine, but they are also driving it to become more patient-centered and an approach much more engaged in medicine, where individuals are taking active participation in the management of their health, empowered with information access and support.

References

Gagneja PS, Gagneja KK (2015) Mobile health (mHealth) technologies. In: 2015 17th international conference on E-health networking, application & services (HealthCom), Boston, MA, USA, pp 37–43. https://doi.org/10.1109/HealthCom.2015.7454470

Ghebrehiwet I, Zaki N, Damseh R et al (2024) Revolutionizing personalized medicine with generative AI: a systematic review. Artif Intell Rev 57:128. https://doi.org/10.1007/s10462-024-10768-5

Hermes S, Riasanow T, Clemons EK et al (2020) The digital transformation of the healthcare industry: exploring the rise of emerging platform ecosystems and their influence on the role of patients. Bus Res 13:1033–1069. https://doi.org/10.1007/s40685-020-00125-x

Jain KK (2021) Development of personalized medicine. In: Textbook of personalized medicine. Springer, Cham. https://doi.org/10.1007/978-3-030-62080-6_22

Kasoju N, Remya NS, Sasi R et al (2023) Digital health: trends, opportunities and challenges in medical devices, pharma and bio-technology. CSIT 11:11–30. https://doi.org/10.1007/s40012-023-00380-3

Lerzynski G (2021) Opening the door for digital transformation in hospitals: management's point of view. In: Glauner P, Plugmann P, Lerzynski G (eds) Digitalization in healthcare. Future of business and finance. Springer, Cham. https://doi.org/10.1007/978-3-030-65896-0_2

Milan L (2023) Artificial intelligence and machine learning in integrated diagnostic. In: Giovanella L (ed) Integrated diagnostics and theranostics of thyroid diseases. Springer, Cham. https://doi.org/10.1007/978-3-031-35213-3_2

Murphy B, Feeney O (2023) AI, data analytics and the professions. In: Lynn T, Rosati P, Conway E, van der Werff L (eds) The future of work. Palgrave studies in digital business & enabling technologies. Palgrave Macmillan, Cham. https://doi.org/10.1007/978-3-031-31494-0_3

Quazi S (2022) Artificial intelligence and machine learning in precision and genomic medicine. Med Oncol 39:120. https://doi.org/10.1007/s12032-022-01711-1

Takahashi M, Koike R, Nagasawa K et al (2022) Development of telemedicine tools with an emphasis on visual observation. Artif Life Robotics 27:38–47. https://doi.org/10.1007/s10015-022-00731-4

Chapter 3
Meta-Health and Its Understanding

3.1 Introduction

The healthcare industry is rapidly embracing the metaverse. The area of healthcare delivery is expected to undergo significant changes due to advancements in AR (augmented reality), VR (virtual reality), AI (artificial intelligence), IoT (Internet of Things), QC (quantum computing), and robotics. In recent times, AR/VR technologies have made significant developments and are now normally employed in surgical procedures and educational and medical training to implement sophisticated surgeries with special accuracy. To improve the usability of medical outfits and bias, these factors are also considered in their software system and problem-solving approaches. Though the metaverse conjures up images of games and entertainment, the underlying technologies are now used in the field of healthcare. These include extended reality (occasionally appertained to as XR or stoked reality, virtual reality, and mixed reality) (Ullah et al. 2023). Blockchain and virtual means are two exemplifications of Web3 technology and operations. M-worlds are real-time virtual "places" where people congregate and produce content. The maturity of healthcare use cases to date uses XR. Innumerable individual and remedial uses, as well as medical education, gatherings, and conferences, all make use of the technology. Blockchain is also being tested by businesses for a variety of uses, including healthcare data operation and force chain verification (Li et al. 2024). The metaverse includes cutting-edge technological inventions like AR, VR, AI, telemedicine, digital twins, and blockchain that have a significant influence on healthcare. By exposing people to new, much less precious remedy delivery styles, these technologies improve patient issues. By the utilization of the Internet, the metaverse simulates mortal conduct and feelings in a virtual terrain. Both the actual world and the virtual world's whole social and profitable structures are involved. Figure 3.1 shows the four axes of the healthcare operations of the metaverse (Gaur and Jhanjhi 2023).

There are several ways that metaverse technology may add value for companies, including the ones listed below:

S. Vyas et al., *Meta-Health*, https://doi.org/10.1007/978-981-96-5844-2_3

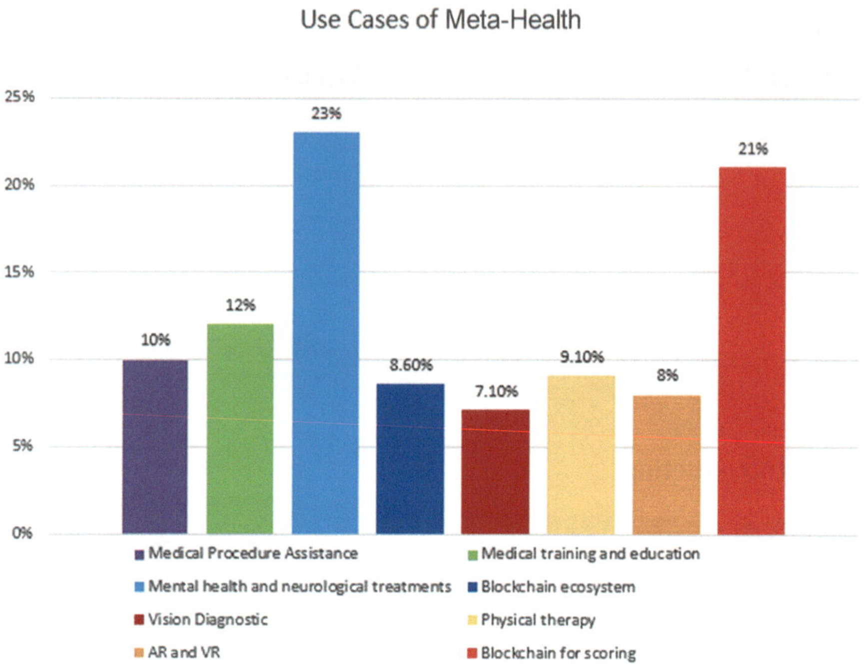

Fig. 3.1 Use cases rates of Meta-Health

- Increasing availability to watch by bridging geographical distances between patients and providers.
- Using cutting-edge technologies to improve the precision of diagnosis and the standard of surgery.
- Creating new opportunities for the storing, distributing, and accessing data (patient, claims, and provider).
- Improving the experience of insurance members and patients.
- Expanding income streams with new offers.
- Reducing operational expenses by simplifying processes including hiring, training, and compensation.

The merging of the metaverse with healthcare enables the virtualization of hundreds of processes, which generates various new paths for the healthcare metaverse, including the following:

1. Mental health and neurological treatments.
2. Rehabilitation and Physical therapy.
3. Medical education and training.
4. Medical procedure assistance.
5. Assistance with medical procedures.
6. The blockchain ecosystem for payments and supply chain applications.

7. The AR/VR infrastructure for biotech.
8. Vision diagnostics and eye tracking.

The use of metaverse technology is already boosting patient's approach to medication, enhancing medical education and training, enhancing conclusions in several diseases and surgical procedure, and sinking costs in numerous ways.

3.2 Emerging Use Cases of Meta-Health

Startups in the healthcare metaverse got more than two billion dollars in private capital throughout the period we researched, with investment growing at a pace of about 35% annually. In addition to supporting the development of enablers and support services (such as medical professionals, healthcare data and analytics, and operations), financing activity was conducted at all phases of the patient experience (patient engagement, care delivery, management, and payment) (Mohammed and Albarrak 2024). Most of the use cases that we found (60% of businesses, 40% of funding) uses XR in some way and pertain to payers or providers. The most active XR-related fields include mental health, medical education, and procedure aid (such as AR-assisted surgery) (Lee 2022). The three areas with the largest financing are medical training, medical procedure help, and infrastructure for AR and VR. Major providers and payers now utilize several of the applications (such as training, mental health, physical therapy, eye diagnostics, and AR-supported surgery). Only 10% of all fundraising dollars are allocated to firms that are developing blockchain technologies, which suggests that the technology is still in its immaturity, and thus smaller funding rounds are being held. Blockchain applications for payers and providers likewise include platforms for sharing and guarding patient data as well as payments (Ullah et al. 2023).

Use cases in metaverse include the following:

- **Telemedicine and Remote Meetings**
  - Virtual treatment center
  - Remote surgery support
- **Medical Education and Training**
  - Virtual medical simulations
  - Improved learning environments
- **Patient Appointment and Therapy**
  - Virtual reality therapy
  - Reducing healthcare anxiety
- **Drug Discovery and Research**
  - Accelerated drug testing
  - Collaborative research in virtual labs

3.3 Technologies for Meta-Health

Figure 3.2 provides an expansive analysis of the essential technologies compelling the application of the metaverse in healthcare. These technologies encompass blockchain, IoT (Internet of Things), AI (artificial intelligence), XR (extended reality), 5G and advanced communication networks, digital binary technology, 3D modeling, big data analytics, computer vision, edge computing, human-computer interaction, and quantum computing (Wang et al. 2022).

1. **XR (Extended Reality)**: Extended reality (XR) incorporates diverse technologies like augmented reality (AR), virtual reality (VR), and mixed reality (MR), all strengthened by AI and associated devices like head-mounted displays, mobile devices, and wearables. By merging voice, motion tracing, gestures, and vision, XR is revolutionizing service delivery and enhancing various sectors' quality. In the healthcare field, the combination of XR and the metaverse holds immense potential. Medical students can now gain practical experience in realistic 3D virtual environments, surpassing the limitations of traditional classrooms. Surgeons, too, can improve their skills through XR applications in the metaverse, enabling them to envisage organs, tumors, X-rays, and ultrasounds in real time from numerous angles during surgeries, thereby increasing efficiency and accelerating treatment. Moreover, in emergencies, the metaverse can guide nonprofessionals through resuscitation procedures, based on simulated environments and XR equipment. Additionally, XR and remote-controlled devices in the metaverse can be utilized for supporting patients with metal therapy, physical therapy, and speech therapy.
2. **Blockchain**: Blockchain is an integral component of the metaverse, as centralized data storage presents security, privacy, and transparency challenges. Embracing blockchain transforms the metaverse into a decentralized digital realm accessible across platforms globally. It eliminates the need for central institutions and enables seamless access to various digital spaces. By incorporating blockchain technology into the metaverse, the process of gathering genuine and valuable data becomes more streamlined. The blockchain's immutability and transparency ensure the secure storage and management of extensive amounts of data within the metaverse.

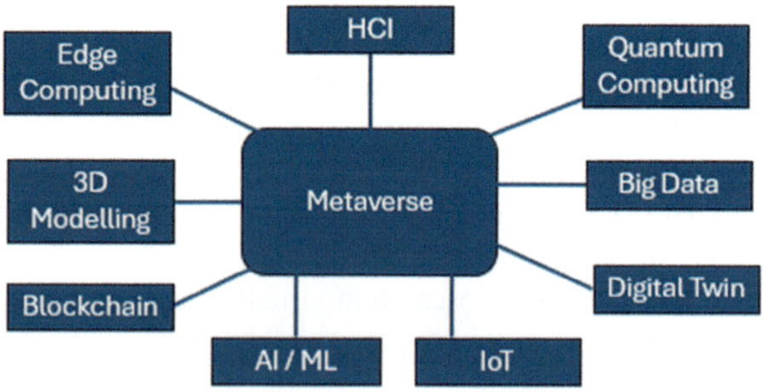

Fig. 3.2 Technologies enabling Meta-Health

3. **Artificial Intelligence**: AI plays a vital role in strengthening the metaverse's organization, improving the 3D immersive capability, and refining virtual world services. Its combination enhances the whole quality of services and the metaverse ecosystem. In the medical field, artificial intelligence (AI) plays a crucial role in analyzing and diagnosing patients' health data. With the aid of AI, the metaverse provides doctors with top-notch 3D images and scans, which are crucial for successful medical interventions. AI also offers valuable insights, assisting in highlighting critical patients and cutting errors in electronic health record (EHR) analysis, resulting in more precise diagnoses. The quick evaluation of electronic health records and biomedical data by artificial intelligence algorithms within the metaverse allows doctors to obtain instant and trustworthy suggestions. Additionally, the collaborative ability of the metaverse and AI presents to fields such as drug discovery, disease forecasting, and emergency response, underscoring the profound impact of this fusion.
4. **Internet of Things (IoT)**: The fusion of the metaverse and the Internet of Things (IoT) will close the gap between the digital and physical domains, ensuing in a more intelligent and reactive world. Remote patient monitoring is one well-known use of this IoT-enabled metaverse in the healthcare industry. Patients can avoid making in-person trips to medical institutions by having their critical health indicators, such as blood pressure, temperature, and heart rate, automatically gathered and displayed by IoT devices in the 3D metaverse environment. Furthermore, surgeons can carry out complex operations that would be difficult for human hands to execute alone thanks to the integration of tiny, Internet-connected nanobots inside the human body that are monitored in the virtual three-dimensional metaverse environment. Smaller incisions result from robotic operations employing IoT devices or nanobots, reducing invasiveness, and accelerating patient recuperation. Furthermore, prospects for managing chronic diseases, better sleep cycles, medication reminders, and timely alerts during health emergencies are presented by the connection between the metaverse and IoT.
5. **Digital Twin**: Digital twins serve as foundational elements of the metaverse, creating digital replicas of every object within it. By determining a digital twin of whole hospital in the metaverse, operational plans, staffing, and care models can be analyzed to meet requirements effectively. In challenging situations such as shortages of bed, pathogen communication, scheduling of doctors, or obtainability of operating rooms, these virtual models in the metaverse can provide valuable insights. Utilizing digital twin technology within the metaverse can enhance patients' treatment, decrease costs, and improve staff performance, making it vital for strategic decision-making in the complex healthcare environment. The complete virtualization of hospitals in the metaverse utilizing digital twins designs a risk-free environment for various applications. Furthermore, the metaverse afforded by digital twins presents potential for the creation of customized artificial organs. Additionally, technology makes it easier to perform virtual simulations of heart and brain surgeries, which allows for practice and improvement prior to attempting complex real-world treatments (Turab and Jamil 2023).

6. **Quantum Computing**: The metaverse tackles important problems with cybersecurity, processing power, and cyberattacks because of quantum computing. As the metaverse grows, quantum-enabled security apps guarantee the essential protection for all healthcare operations and transactions. By utilizing the enormous computational power of quantum computing, healthcare applications in the metaverse become more efficient and gain better simulation and computation processes. As a result of this development, connections between medical professionals and patients using the metaverse's healthcare applications are improved overall. The incorporation of quantum computing into the metaverse not only solves problems but opens revolutionary possibilities for safe and effective healthcare delivery. The metaverse's quantum computing capabilities have enormous potential to influence healthcare in the future.
7. **3D Modelling**: Replicating real-world things in 3D within the metaverse's virtual environment is crucial to its success. The 3D modeling capabilities of the metaverse are essential in the healthcare industry. Making educated selections about their purchases is made easier for patients by providing them with 3D views of medical products and interactive anatomical representations. Medical professionals can better grasp their patients' conditions, thanks to the metaverse's 3D modeling, which enables them to administer more accurate diagnoses and treatments. Medical researchers can also apply the metaverse's 3D modeling experiences to build artificial organs and estimate their functioning in various simulated situations. This has a tremendous deal of promise to advance medical innovation and research. In the end, 3D replication expertise within the metaverse greatly improves patient experiences and results.

3.4 Meta-Health Framework for Healthcare

Nowadays, digital experiences generally concentrate on information access via transactional means. Conversely, the metaverse is conceived to enable immersive engagements such as learning, purchasing, healthcare delivery, and many more that minimizes the gap between real-life and virtual connections. The huge potential of the metaverse has seen significant investment and interest from major tech firms who are introducing initiatives that blur the line between physical and digital worlds. To have any chance of success, an interoperable ecosystem must be created so that different immersive technologies can be seamlessly integrated. This will encompass emerging technologies like AR, VR, XR, AI, IoT, and 5G as well as scalable and secure computing environments. With the advent of metaverse, people will engage in a new era of interconnection that will change how they interact with others or take part in various activities beyond just digital transactions.

Figure 3.3 is of a healthcare-based version of Jon Radoff's "The seven layers of the metaverse" which highlights the need to solidify infrastructural technologies before branching out into a full-blown virtual world. The Meta-Health includes six vital parts that merge superior basic technologies, AI-empowered interactions, and

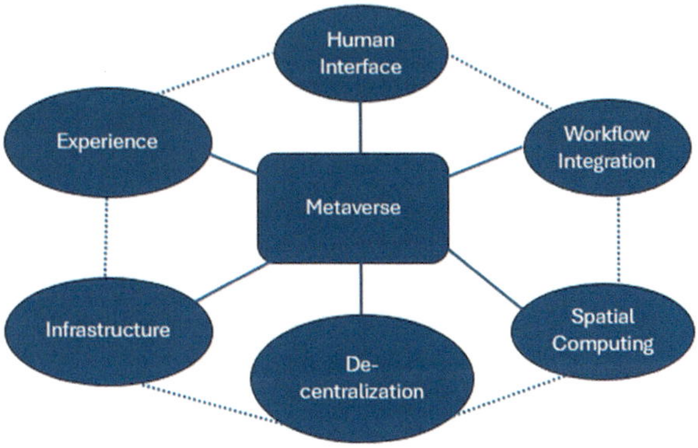

Fig. 3.3 The seven layers of the metaverse

spatial computing in all customer connections. This blend aspires to provide engaging services that possess an intimate touch with each customer, be it in real life or metaverse. For instance, robust technology development must be prioritized when creating a strong medical environment within virtual realms.

3.5 Making of Meta-Health: Approaches for the Metaverse Service Advancement in the Healthcare Industry

- **Healthcare Learning and Training Strategy**: Regarding healthcare education, the strategy directs on incorporating metaverse applications to suit the era of no face to face. This means investigating how Objective Structured Clinical Examination (OSCE) and clinical performance evaluation (CPX) could be carried out with meta-human, switching simulation-based patients that were traditionally used. The aim is to improve the quality of healthcare education by using metaverse technology, while developing highly competent professionals with master's or doctorate degrees in health industries specialized in metaverse.
- **Strategy of Deploying Metaverse Technology in Healthcare**: As a result of this, the approach is intended to maximize the role of metaverse technology in solving many healthcare challenges. This will necessitate using the benefits of technologies used in other sectors to make significant changes into healthcare. The most crucial point here is laying down an investment base for metaverse adoption across all regions thereby lessening the digital divide in healthcare. At the same time, launching initiatives such as metaverse Fund would attract private investments into healthcare industry before addressing ethical issues that emerge from metaverse health services.
- **Advancement of Healthcare Business Environment Strategy**: The main thrust of this strategy is to enhance the healthcare service environment through a variety of mechanisms. This includes support for basic technology and finished products for healthcare devices. Another key milestone is the creation of a

comprehensive metaverse data repository for large clinical and nonclinical data in the healthcare industry. Develop and promote health services initiatives suitable for metaverse environments.

- **Provision for Ensuring Global Competitions in Healthcare Strategy**: This strategy is focused around securing worldwide competitiveness in the healthcare industry. It implies encouraging healthcare unicorn businesses through intensive support to drive innovation and growth. Additionally, the strategy focuses on securing future innovative technologies specifically tailored for the healthcare industry, like metaverse technology visualization. To bolster international presence, metaverse corporate globalization will be actively promoted. In formulation for borderless interactions among clinics, consumers, doctors, and patients, the strategy will also entail the development of metaverse promotion laws and major regulations (Farahat et al. 2023).

3.6 Healthcare Industries Working on Metaverse

- **Latus Healthcare**: Latus Healthcare is currently working on the creation of a cutting-edge "virtual hospital" that will exist in a virtual reality environment. The main aim of this healthcare company is to provide physiotherapy facilities. By taking advantage of the abilities of VR, Latus Healthcare intends to deliver advanced and immersive medications to patients, transforming the way physiotherapy is performed.
- **iMining**: iMining is set to make history by establishing the world's first ever Hospital Foundation in the Decentraland Metaverse. This innovative system will open new frontiers in healthcare, allowing users to access treatments and information in the virtual realm. Leveraging the power of the Decentraland platform, iMining aims to redefine the concept of accessing and delivering healthcare services, allowing users to interact with healthcare resources in innovative and interactive ways.
- **Apollo Hospitals**: In a new development, Apollo Hospitals has now announced its landmark association with "8chili Inc." for engagement in the metaverse. This would bring together the medical expertise of Apollo Hospitals and the technology prowess of "8chili Inc." in what could emerge as some never-before kind of healthcare experience created in virtual settings. This aims to merge medical knowledge with capabilities offered by the metaverse so that interactions and simulations can improve treatment provided to patients, education among doctors, and research activities.

In summary, these three enterprises highlight the expanding relevance of healthcare and the metaverse. From Latus Healthcare's virtual clinic offering fitness services in a virtual reality environment to the pioneering iMining foundation in the Decentraland metaverse, and the Apollo Clinics with "8chili Inc." to join the metaverse, the healthcare industry is embracing the potential of virtual realms to change patient acceptance and experiences. These initiatives demonstrate efforts to expand future treatment possibilities by integrating cutting-edge technology into healthcare.

3.7 Future Consequences of Meta-Health

- **Virtual Hospitals on the Rise**: The emergence of virtual hospitals means the creation of a virtual environment that simulates an atmosphere of a medical setting accessed through headsets mainly offering counselling and physiotherapy services; new technologies are utilized during physiotherapy, such as computer vision which evaluates the extent of recovery achieved by patients and degree of motion in injured joints. The concept is being explored aggressively by Latus Healthcare of the UK, which is developing a virtual hospital and plans to run this service within the next 12–18 months. In a most enterprising move, Apollo Hospitals Group of India has tied up with 8chili Inc. to expand into the metaverse with a virtual hospital. Virtual reality in the metaverse, as a tool of patient counseling, puts a patient into calming environments to give them power to take over and control their physiology for emotional self-regulation and regulation to increase patient satisfaction (Chengoden et al. 2023).
- **Gamification in Healthcare**: Games have been widely used in health and wellness interventions targeting disease prevention, medication observance, telemedicine, and self-management. By emphasizing patient-centeredness, health gaming aims to validate patient experiences and increase engagement. Metaverse provides an ideal platform to improve this process, providing patients with a participatory virtual environment to complete tasks and challenges, and earn rewards such as badges that allow patients to set their own goals and they compete with others, motivating them to remain involved in their healthcare activities. Examples include US-based Mango Health, which promotes timely medication compliance and bonuses patients with badges, and the Happify platform, which provides science-based activities to enhance emotional well-being.
- **AR/VR Empowered Surgeries**: Multimodal applications of augmented reality (AR) in healthcare include areas such as behavioral healthcare, diagnostic imaging, surgical procedures, etc. It is anticipated that health surgery industry will see a dramatic increase in AR/VR adoption, with market forecasts reaching $16.2 billion by 2027. This advanced technology plays an important role in preoperative planning, training, and procedures approach to diagnosis. Leading companies such as Immersive Touch and EchoPixel in the United States have developed AR/VR platforms for detailed patient-specific physical examination and virtual surgical planning (Lakshmi et al. 2024; Musamih et al. 2022).
- **Advancements in Medical Education and Training**: Metaverse adds significant value to medical education by facilitating interactive learning and simulation training. Unlike traditional single channel virtual school courses, metaverse enables students to interact with each other in online clinical courses and simulations. Medical training in the metaverse proves particularly effective for

complex procedures that require advanced hands-on skills and communication skills. Platforms like Metamedix VR in the European Union are creating 3D virtual environments for medical training, allowing doctors and nurses to train anywhere and democratizing access to treatments and programs around the world. Additionally, Veyond metaverse in the USA connects healthcare professionals around the world in collaborative education, training, and medical activities and uses the cloud and state-of-the-art real-time communication technologies to enhance clinician skills (Musamih et al. 2022).

References

Chengoden R, Victor N, Huynh-The T, Yenduri G, Jhaveri RH, Alazab M et al (2023) Metaverse for healthcare: a survey on potential applications, challenges and future directions. IEEE Access 11:12765–12795

Farahat MA, Darwish A, Hassanien AE (2023) The implication of metaverse in the traditional medical environment and healthcare sector: applications and challenges. In: Hassanien AE, Darwish A, Torky M (eds) The future of metaverse in the virtual era and physical world. Studies in big data, vol 123. Springer, Cham. https://doi.org/10.1007/978-3-031-29132-6_7

Gaur L, Jhanjhi NZ (eds) (2023) Metaverse applications for intelligent healthcare. IGI Global, Hershey

Lakshmi D, Kondurkar I, Kumar R, Banerjee R (2024) Intelligent healthcare systems in the metaverse: architecture, applications, challenges, and opportunities. In: The metaverse for the healthcare industry. Springer, Berlin, pp 17–32

Lee CW (2022) Application of metaverse service to healthcare industry: a strategic perspective. Int J Environ Res Public Health 19(20):13038

Li Y, Gunasekeran DV, RaviChandran N, Tan TF, Ong JCL, Thirunavukarasu AJ et al (2024) The next generation of healthcare ecosystem in the metaverse. Biom J 47(3):100679

Mohammed R, Albarrak A (2024) The use of metaverse in the health-care system: a scoping review article. Hail J Health Sci 6(1):24–30

Musamih A, Yaqoob I, Salah K, Jayaraman R, Al-Hammadi Y, Omar M, Ellahham S (2022) Metaverse in healthcare: applications, challenges, and future directions. IEEE Consumer Electron Mag 12(4):33–46

Turab M, Jamil S (2023) A comprehensive survey of digital twins in healthcare in the era of metaverse. BioMedInformatics 3(3):563–584

Ullah H, Manickam S, Obaidat M, Laghari SUA, Uddin M (2023) Exploring the potential of metaverse technology in healthcare: applications, challenges, and future directions. IEEE Access 11:69686–69707

Wang G, Badal A, Jia X, Maltz JS, Mueller K, Myers KJ et al (2022) Development of metaverse for intelligent healthcare. Nat Mach Intell 4(11):922–929

Chapter 4
Technologies Enabling Meta-Health

4.1 Introduction

The theory of the metaverse, once narrowed to the fields of science fiction, is now materializing into a dynamical, immersive virtual world with widespread associations across diverse industries. In healthcare, the metaverse signifies a new frontier, blending digital and physical realities to create a range of care that develops ahead of the conventional boundaries of hospitals. This merging is made feasible by a collection of advanced technologies that jointly build and assist the metaverse, converting how healthcare is served, retrieved, and qualified.

The core of the metaverse are technologies like artificial intelligence (AI), virtual reality (VR), augmented reality (AR), blockchain, and the Internet of Things (IoT) as shown in Fig. 4.1. These innovations are not only improving presented healthcare methods but also flagging the way for completely new modes of patient interface, medical training, and research.

AR and VR have unlocked new avenues for healthcare professionals to involve with patients and train in simulated situations that meticulously mimic real-life setups. Doctors can now operate difficult processes in virtual settings, while medical scholars can learn in extremely collaborative, risk-free conditions. AI is portraying a gradually more critical role by managing vast amounts of data to aid in diagnostics, planning, and specified medicine, thus upgrading patient results and operating proficiency.

Blockchain confirms the security and integrity of health data, focusing established concerns about data breaches and privacy. This distributed approach to data management not only advances enormous trust between patients and practitioners but also assists unified sharing of information within different stages in the metaverse. IoT facilitates real-time examining and data collection, improving patient care by catering constant, actionable perceptions (Mohammed and Albarrak 2024).

As these technologies come together, they are not without challenges. Ethical consequences, data privacy, and the digital division are significant concerns that

S. Vyas et al., *Meta-Health*, https://doi.org/10.1007/978-981-96-5844-2_4

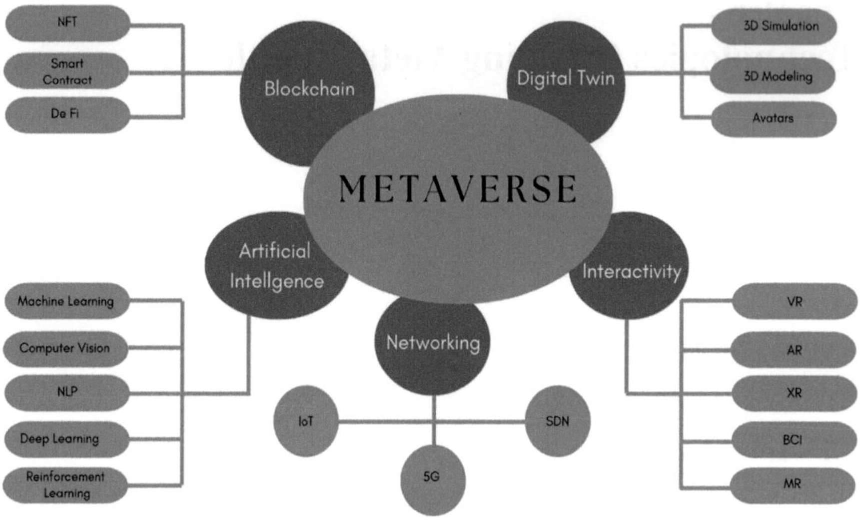

Fig. 4.1 Technologies enabling metaverse

need to be tackled to ensure impartial access and safe implementation of metaverse-enabled healthcare resolutions. Also, regulatory frameworks will need to evolve to keep speed with the rapid technological innovations and to provide transparent recommendations for their treatment in healthcare (Chengoden et al. 2023).

4.2 Technologies Shaping Meta-Health

4.2.1 Wearable Health Devices

In the always changing environment of healthcare, wearable health gadgets have emerged as innovative devices that offer new insights into personal health and well-being. These devices encompass a range of technology, from biosensors to smartwatches, and have transitioned from accessories to being essential tools used to monitor health metrics and vital signs. Wearable technology is the result of embedding sophisticated sensors, design, and networking technology into everyday accessories. The close-to-body nature of wearable technology means that people can now be monitored continuously for a variety of physiological measures and health indices. The wearables of today have such a wide range of features including physical activity tracking, measure of heart rate, sleep analysis, and stress management, in part due to developing sensor technology and advancements in the field of nanotechnology (Baggam and Rani 2025).

Wearable Health Device Examples: The wearable health devices currently on the market are assorted products aimed to address different health needs. Well-known examples include smartwatches with heart rate monitors, accelerometers, and global positioning system (GPS) capabilities, which are now able to track physical activity levels and provide real-time data feedback about their health goals. Wearable biosensors, such as Continuous Glucose Monitors (CGM) and Electrocardiogram (ECG) monitors, have progressively transformed the way chronic disease is managed, not only because they provide patients with practical data on their health status but also regarding what technology is now available in such a small device.

Role in Monitoring Health Parameters and Vital Signs: Some of the prime applications of wearable health devices are in tracking health parameters and vital signs. Such devices, aided by a mixture of sensors and data analytics, provide a glimpse of the summary view on the physiological status of a user, thereby allowing for the detection of irregularities at an early stage and proactive management of health concerns. For example, wearable ECG monitors can detect an arrhythmia and warn the user to seek help prior to a potentially fatal event.

Several opportunities and challenges exist for wearable health devices in their attempt at changing healthcare delivery. One of the big hurdles concerns the privacy issues of collecting and using personal health information. Tight data security measures will, therefore, be essential, as well as clear directions about privacy. Moreover, the accuracy and reliability of wearable sensors present persistent challenges that require them to undergo continuous validation and calibration in their provision of accuracy for health monitoring. With developments in artificial intelligence, data analytics, and sensor technologies, wearable health devices are poised to have a bright future. The dissemination of these technologies will certainly change the health setting into one that permits people to live a healthier life and advances a more active method to manage the health. Additionally, by means of artificial intelligence algorithms, the ability of wearables will be enhanced to provide better, timely, and tailored interventions for user needs and prediction of health events. The significant module of Meta-Health Wearable sensor technology brings in a new age for individualized, data-driven healthcare. There is a future where healthcare is not just preventive and proactive but is really personalized according to the different needs of each individual and is proactive on the wearable technology front (Mohammed and Albarrak 2024).

4.2.2 Artificial Intelligence in Healthcare

In the Meta-Health paradigm, with a focus on holistic, personalized healthcare over disease-centric models, AI plays a critical role in obtaining insights from massive health datasets to inform decision-making. One of the more visible applications of AI in Meta-Health is predictive analytics, wherein machine learning algorithms are examined through electronic health records, genomic data, and routine data for trends that can predict which individuals are at risk for specific health conditions.

With these insights in place, preemptive healthcare is possible, giving a person-centric view of preventive methods and interventions at least in part based on the risk profile (Wang et al. 2022).

AI-powered diagnostics has transformed the way diseases are detected and diagnosed today with high accuracy and efficiency. Machine learning algorithms trained on voluminous datasets of medical images can pick up very minute and subtle abnormalities and disease patterns, thereby facilitating early detection and intervention. Besides that, artificial intelligence-powered clinical decision support systems help health providers devise treatment plans tailored towards the data of a particular patient for optimizing the medicinal outcome and decreasing adverse effects.

Although AI has obvious advantages in Meta-Health, its pervasive diffusion is raising several ethical concerns and challenges. First and foremost is the accountability of AI algorithms and transparency in critical decision-making processes such as diagnosis and treatment planning. It is for the developers of AI-driven healthcare solutions to ensure fairness and equity toward avoiding algorithmic biases and disparities in patient outcomes. Moreover, the ethical management of patient information on privacy concerns and security of data calls for very strong regulatory frameworks and ethical guidelines to ensure that the rights of patients and confidentiality are observed.

Although AI algorithms progress and learn from varied data sources, they will become progressively expert at predicting disease trails, recognizing optimal treatment approaches, and individualizing healthcare involvements. Moreover, the integration of AI with such emerging technologies as wearable health devices or telemedicine platforms will expand its scope and influence on uniform remote monitoring and care delivery.

Successfully capturing the potential of AI in Meta-Health and applying it to practice will require vigorous efforts to surmount many technical, ethical, and regulatory challenges. In this respect, constructing transparent and accountable AI solutions that clearly make patient safety, privacy, and equity a priority will call for collaboration from all stakeholders in the healthcare sector, technology developers, policymakers, and ethicists. Furthermore, investment in education and workforce development related to AI is important to ensure that healthcare professionals acquire relevant skills and competencies needed for the successful application of AI in clinical practice.

4.2.3 Remote Patient Monitoring and Telemedicine

Telemedicine may be defined as the delivery of healthcare at a distance using telecommunications technology for consultation, diagnosis, and treatment. The concept of telemedicine evolved over the last several decades, catalyzed by new and improved telecommunications infrastructure, digital health technologies, and evolving models for healthcare delivery. From simple telephone consultations, it has evolved into video conferencing, mobile health apps, and out-of-reach monitoring devices that allow healthcare providers to deliver quality care to patients irrespective of the geographical boundaries. RPM technologies permit healthcare providers to track the patient's health status and vital signs remotely, often in real-time, with the use of wearable devices, sensors, and mobile health applications.

These are innovations that advance the concept of constant observation of physiological parameters, such as blood pressure, pulse, glucose levels, and activity levels, to facilitate early detection of wellness issues and proactive intervention. Furthermore, RPM empowers patients to actively participate in their own care and enables them to make informed decisions regarding their health and wellness (Mohammed and Albarrak 2024).

In the advent of Meta-Health, characterized by the flagship agendas of personalization and comprehensive care, telemedicine and remote monitoring hold a variety of advantages. First is that they open new avenues for healthcare providers to extend treatment as per the requirement of an individual irrespective of his geographical location or the nature of physical disability he/she may be afflicted with. Even access to specialist consultations, chronic disease management, and preventive health services can be accorded to the patients in the comfort zone of their homes, reducing the travel burden and thus enhancing convenience. Furthermore, telemedicine and remote monitoring facilitate the proactive management of health conditions by allowing for early intervention and preventing complications. Because the well-being status and trends of patients are tracked continuously, a healthcare provider can identify any possible problems before surging, reducing hospitalization, emergency office visits, and consequently the costs of healthcare (Farahat et al. 2023). Moreover, telemedicine improves access to care for underserved populations, such as rural communities, elderly persons, and those with limited mobility, thereby bridging gaps in healthcare disparities and advancing healthcare value.

Whereas telemedicine and inaccessible understanding observation hold enormous promises, they raise administrative and legitimate considerations that must be attended to in a manner that will ensure secure and effective application. Regulatory frameworks around licensure, repayment, protection, and security differ across domains and healthcare settings, hence testing far-reaching reception and consolidation into clinical practice. Furthermore, lawful concerns like risk, educated assent, and misbehavior securities require careful attention to alleviate dangers and secure both patients and healthcare suppliers.

The future for telemedicine and deeper understanding in checking is bright, powered by progressing progressions in advanced well-being advances, manufactured insights, and networks. In the future of telemedicine, progressing stages will end up progressively coordination with electronic healthcare records, information analytics, and AI-driven clinical choice bolster frameworks that can administer nonstop, personalized care conveyance. In addition, the expansion of wearable gadgets and Internet of Things (IoT) sensors will advance the scope of farther observing and encouraging persistent, real-time following of patients' healthcare status and behaviors. Be that as it may, realizing the total potential of telemedicine and farther observing requires tending to tireless challenges related to administrative, legal, and repayment boundaries. Policymakers and controllers must collaborate with partners to create standardized rules, interoperable frameworks, and repayment models that incentivize the selection of telemedicine and inaccessible checking whereas guaranteeing understanding security and security. Also, ventures in advanced foundation, broadband get to, and computerized proficiency programs are fundamental to bridge the computerized isolate and guarantee impartial get to telemedicine administrations for all populaces (Sujatha et al. 2025).

4.2.4 Big Data Analytics for Health Insights

Enormous information analytics alludes to the method of analyzing huge and complex datasets to reveal designs, patterns, and bits of knowledge that can illuminate decision-making and drive significant results. Within the setting of healthcare, enormous information analytics includes the accumulation and examination of assorted sources of healthcare information, counting electronic healthcare records, genomic information, restorative imaging, wearable gadget information, and populace healthcare information. By tackling progressed analytics procedures such as machine learning, information mining, and prescient modeling, enormous information analytics empowers healthcare organizations to determine profitable experiences, optimize clinical workflows, and move forward persistent results.

Within the period of Meta-Health, where the center shifts from receptive malady administration to proactive, personalized care, enormous information plays an essential part in opening the complete potential of healthcare information. By joining and analyzing tremendous sums of differing healthcare information, counting clinical, hereditary, natural, and way of life components, enormous information analytics empowers a comprehensive understanding of individuals' healthcare status, hazard variables, and treatment reactions. This all-encompassing approach to data-driven healthcare enables healthcare suppliers to convey personalized intercessions custom-made to everyone's interesting needs, subsequently optimizing healthcare results and upgrading, in general, the quality of care.

Enormous information analytics includes a wide run of applications over different spaces of healthcare, counting clinical care, investigation, populace healthcare administration, and healthcare operations. In clinical care, enormous information analytics empowers prescient modeling of malady directions, early location of unfavorable occasions, and optimization of treatment techniques through accuracy pharmaceutical approaches. In the investigation, enormous information analytics encourages speculation era, recognize proof of biomarkers, and sedate disclosure by analyzing large-scale genomic, proteomic, and clinical datasets. In populace healthcare administration, huge information analytics bolsters chance stratification and malady reconnaissance and focuses on intercessions to improve healthcare results at the community level. Also, in healthcare operations, enormous information analytics improves effectiveness, asset allotment, and income optimization by analyzing operational data, patient stream designs, and healthcare utilization patterns.

Whereas enormous information analytics holds gigantic guarantee in healthcare, it too raises critical protection and security concerns related to the collection, capacity, and utilization of delicate healthcare information. The accumulation of differing datasets containing individual healthcare data (PHI) postured dangers of information breaches, unauthorized get to, and abuse of information, possibly compromising quiet security and secrecy. Additionally, the anonymization and de-identification of healthcare information may not continuously ensure privacy protection, as propels in re-identification techniques posture challenges to information anonymization strategies. Also, compliance with administrative systems such as the Healthcare Insurance Portability and Responsibility Act (HIPAA) and the Common Information Security Direction (GDPR) requires healthcare organizations to actualize vigorous information security measures, security shields, and assent instruments to ensure quiet rights and moderate security dangers related with huge information analytics.

Looking ahead, the long run of huge information analytics in healthcare holds huge guarantee, driven by continuous headways in data science, counterfeit insights, and advanced healthcare advances. As healthcare organizations proceed to digitize their operations and receive electronic healthcare records (EHRs), the volume and assortment of healthcare information accessible for investigation will proceed to develop exponentially, showing modern openings for inferring noteworthy bits of knowledge and driving advancement in healthcare conveyance.

In addition, the integration of enormous information analytics with rising advances such as wearable gadgets, telemedicine stages, and IoT sensors will assist in extending the scope of data-driven healthcare, empowering nonstop, real-time checking of individuals' healthcare status and behaviors. By leveraging prescient modeling and AI-driven calculations, healthcare suppliers can expect healthcare dangers, personalize interventions, and engage people to take proactive control of their healthcare and well-being.

Be that as it may, realizing the complete potential of enormous information analytics in healthcare requires tending to tireless challenges related to information interoperability, information quality, and information administration. Collaborative endeavors between healthcare organizations, innovation sellers, policymakers, and administrative organizations are basic to create standardized information trade conventions, interoperable information platforms, and administration systems that encourage consistent sharing and examination of healthcare data while safeguarding understanding protection and secrecy.

4.2.5 Blockchain in Healthcare

Blockchain innovation could be a decentralized, conveyed record framework that empowers secure and straightforward record-keeping of exchanges across an organized network of computers. Each square within the blockchain contains a cryptographic hash of the past piece, making an unchanging chain of information that is safe to altering or unauthorized adjustment. Through agreement instruments such as confirmation of work or verification of stake, blockchain guarantees the keenness and dependability of information without requiring for middle people or central specialists.

In healthcare, blockchain innovation holds gigantic guarantee intending to longstanding challenges related to information interoperability, security, and keenness. One of the key applications of blockchain is the secure capacity and sharing of electronic healthcare records (EHRs), empowering patients to preserve control over their individual healthcare data and allow get to healthcare suppliers as required. Similarly, blockchain advances the secure trade of medicinal information amid discrete frameworks, rationalizing care matching and allowing uniform progression of care over healthcare situations.

During the time of Meta-Health, in which individual and integrative care is relevant, blockchain offers a few advantages that adjust according to the standards of transparency, security, and quiet empowerment. Blockchain advances belief and truthfulness in healthcare through a tamper-resistant record of well-being information interactions, thus cultivating collaborative decision-making between patients and healthcare practitioners. Moreover, blockchain gives patients a secure way of sharing well-being information with analysts to contribute toward the progression of restorative information and advancement of customized treatment procedures.

Even with its promising advantages, the extended adoption of blockchain in healthcare is sure to run into several implementation barriers. Interoperability is a big step, as many of these healthcare frameworks were anchored on variable rules and standards of information exchange. Besides, scalability, performance, and other compliance issues will have to be overcome for blockchain solutions to have a practical, viable place in healthcare settings. In any case, activities such as consortia, benchmarks/improvement of organizations, and administrative systems are rising to address these challenges and encourage the appropriation of blockchain innovation in healthcare.

Looking ahead, end of the blockchain in healthcare holds massive guarantee, driven by progressing headways in innovation, administrative systems, and industry collaboration. As blockchain arrangements proceed to develop and advance, they will end up progressively directing into existing healthcare foundation, empowering consistent information trade and interoperability across healthcare systems. Additionally, the integration of blockchain with rising innovations such as fake insights, Web of Things (WoT), and decentralized fund (DeFi) will advance its applications and affect changes in healthcare results. To realize the full potential of blockchain in healthcare, partners must proceed to collaborate and enhance, tending to specialize, administrative, and social barriers to adoption. Activities such as pilot ventures, proof of concepts, and industry associations are basic to illustrate the esteem and possibility of blockchain arrangements in real-world healthcare situations.

4.2.6 Augmented Reality and Virtual Reality in Healthcare

Expanded reality (AR) and virtual reality (VR) are immersive innovations that mix the advanced and physical universes, advertising intelligently and immersive encounters to clients. AR overlays advanced data onto the genuine world, improving discernment and interaction with the environment, whereas VR makes completely virtual situations, transporting clients to mimicked universes. In healthcare, AR and VR have developed as effective devices for therapeutic preparing, understanding instruction, surgical arranging, and recovery, revolutionizing the way we see, connected with, and provide healthcare administrations. AR and VR innovations offer unparalleled openings for therapeutic preparing and instruction, giving immersive, hands-on encounters to restorative understudies, inhabitants, and healthcare experts. VR-based therapeutic recreations allow trainees the practice of surgical techniques, clinical scenarios, and sustained judgment in a hands-on, risk-free manner, developing proficiency and confidence. AR-based anatomical models and educational applications are likely to improve understanding of complex anatomical structures and therapeutic concepts and promote intuitive learning experiences beyond conventional lecture readings and presentations. AR and VR innovations in surgical planning and recovery provide fundamental tools to enhance the accuracy, efficiency, and comprehension of outcomes. AR-assisted surgical navigation systems merge preoperative imaging information with the patient's life structures in real time, providing specialists with upgraded visualization and guidance during complex strategies. It allows patients to lock in VR-based restoration programs that offer individualized and immersive treatment sessions targeting specific motor skills, cognitive abilities, and mental health in attempts to promote recoveries and improvements in the quality of life.

As the advances of AR and VR ended up more open and reasonable, they will become increasingly organized into clinical workflows, restorative instruction educational module, and quiet care pathways. Increased reality will empower healthcare suppliers to get to real-time clinical data, visualize complex restorative information, and associate with computerized substance within the setting of the patient's environment, improving clinical decision-making, and understanding results. VR will proceed to convert therapeutic preparing, simulation-based instruction, and restorative mediations, advertising immersive, personalized encounters that optimize learning, execution, and restoration. From surgical recreations and procedural preparing to torment administration and mental healthcare treatment,

AR and VR will revolutionize the way we convey healthcare administrations, enabling patients and healthcare providers to attain superior results and improve quality of life.

To realize the complete potential of AR and VR in healthcare, partners must collaborate to address specialized, administrative, and moral considerations. Ventures inquire about advancement, and usage is needed to fasten the development and guarantee the security, adequacy, and rationality of AR and VR solutions. By saddling the control of immersive advances, we could change healthcare delivery, improve understanding encounters, and shape a future where personalized, intuitive care is the standard.

4.2.7 Genomics and Personalized Medicine

Genomics alludes to the consideration of an organism's total set of DNAs, counting all its qualities and inherited fabric. Personalized medication, moreover, known as exactness pharmaceutical, utilizes data approximately an individual's hereditary cosmetics, together with other variables such as the way of life and environment, to tailor restorative treatment and avoidance procedures to their one-of-a-kind characteristics. By leveraging experiences from genomics, personalized pharmaceutical points to optimize persistent results, minimize antagonistic effects, and move forward the proficiency of healthcare mediations. Within the period of Meta-Health, where the center shifts from disease-centric to all-encompassing, personalized healthcare, genomics, and personalized pharmaceutical play a significant part in forming preventive procedures and optimizing well-being results. By analyzing an individual's hereditary inclinations, healthcare suppliers can recognize people at higher hazard for certain infections and execute focused medications to avoid or delay their onset. Additionally, personalized pharmaceutical empowers the customization of treatment plans based on hereditary components, maximizing viability and minimizing antagonistic impacts.

Despite its potential benefits, the far-reaching appropriation of personalized medication faces a few challenges that must be addressed to realize its full potential. One of the essential challenges is the complexity and fetching of genomic testing and examination, which may restrain availability and reasonableness for certain populations. Moreover, joining genomic information into clinical decision-making forms requires a strong bioinformatics foundation, intriguing collaboration, and continuous instruction and preparation for healthcare suppliers. Additionally, moral and social contemplations, such as protection, assent, and the even-handed conveyance of benefits and dangers, must be carefully tended to guarantee that personalized medication is executed reasonably and dependably. Besides, administrative systems overseeing the utilization of hereditary information, counting issues related to information protection, informed consent, and hereditary separation, require cautious thought to ensure persistent rights and guarantee the moral conduct of inquiring about and clinical hone.

Genomics and personalized medication speak to effective instruments within the time of Meta-Health, empowering a move towards more exact, personalized, and preventive healthcare methodologies. By leveraging experiences from an individual's hereditary cosmetics, healthcare suppliers can tailor intercessions to their one-of-a-kind characteristics, optimizing treatment results and progressing patient experiences. In any case, realizing the total potential of personalized pharmaceuticals requires tending to critical challenges related to openness, reasonableness, information protection, and moral contemplation. By cultivating collaboration between stakeholders and contributing to inquiries about instruction and foundation, we will tackle the control of genomics and personalized medication to revolutionize healthcare conveyance, improve quiet results, and shape a future where healthcare is personalized, preventive, and patient centric.

Furthermore, long-term genomics and personalized medication hold monstrous guarantees, driven by continuous progressions in innovation, investigation, and clinical honing. As genomic sequencing advances become more reasonable and open, the utilization of hereditary data in clinical decision-making will become progressively common in different healthcare settings. Additionally, the integration of genomics with other "omics" innovations, such as proteomics and metabolomics, will empower a more comprehensive understanding of illness instruments and personalized treatment reactions. Also, headways in manufactured intelligence and machine learning calculations will upgrade our capacity to decipher and analyze large-scale genomic datasets, encouraging the revelation of novel biomarkers, helpful targets, and prescient models for malady chance and treatment reactions.

4.2.8 Nanotechnology in Healthcare

Nanotechnology includes the control of materials at the nanoscale, regularly extending from 1 to 100 nm in measure. At this scale, materials display special physical, chemical, and natural properties that can be tackled for a wide extend of applications, including healthcare. Nanotechnology has revolutionized different viewpoints of healthcare, from medicate conveyance and imaging to diagnostics and regenerative pharmaceuticals, advertising exceptional exactness and effectiveness within the discovery, treatment, and administration of infections. Nanotechnology has enabled noteworthy progressions within the conclusion and treatment of different illnesses, advertising focused on the conveyance of helpful specialists and upgraded imaging capabilities. Nanoparticle-based medicate conveyance frameworks, such as liposomes and polymeric nanoparticles, empower exact control over sedate discharge energy, making strides in restorative adequacy and minimizing antagonistic impacts. Furthermore, nanoparticle-based imaging operators, such as quantum specks and gold nanoparticles, upgrade the affectability and specificity of therapeutic imaging modalities, empowering early detection and exact determination of diseases (Elabiad 2025).

Within the period of Meta-Health, where personalized, data-driven healthcare is fundamental, nanomedicine holds a gigantic guarantee in optimizing persistent results and upgrading the quality of life. By leveraging the one-of-a-kind properties of nanomaterials, nanomedicine empowers the advancement of personalized treatment procedures custom-made to a person's understanding of characteristics, such as hereditary cosmetics, illness arrangement, and physiological parameters. Besides, nanomedicine encourages a focus on the delivery of restorative operators to cells or tissues, maximizing helpful viability and minimizing systemic harmfulness, in this manner moving forward persistent encounters and treatment results.

Whereas nanotechnology offers huge potential in healthcare, its far-reaching appropriation faces few challenges that must be addressed to realize its full benefits. One of the essential challenges is the translation of nanomedicine from seat to bedside, counting issues related to adaptability, fabricating, and administrative approval. Additionally, concerns concerning the security, biocompatibility, and long-term impacts of nanomaterials on human well-being must be completely examined to guarantee the security and viability of nanomedicine in clinical hone. Besides, moral and societal contemplations, such as impartial get to nanomedicine, reasonableness, and persistent assent, require cautious consideration to guarantee that nanotechnology benefits all populaces and adjusts with moral standards of healthcare conveyance. Despite these challenges, continuous headways in nanotechnology, coupled with intriguing collaboration and speculation in inquiries about and improvement, hold the potential to overcome obstructions and open the total potential of nanomedicine in revolutionizing healthcare delivery, making strides in understanding results, and forming a future where healthcare is genuinely personalized, preventive, and patient centered (Mazumdar et al. 2025).

4.3 Ethical, Legal, and Social Implications of Meta-Health Technologies

As Meta-Health innovations proceed to advance, it is important to address moral contemplations encompassing their improvement, utilization, and development. These considerations incorporate ensuring persistent independence, protection, and refined approval in information collection, capacity, and sharing. Besides, healthcare experts must maintain standards of advantage guaranteeing that technology-driven negotiations prioritize understanding well-being and minimize potential hurts. Truthfulness, responsibility, and rationality are fundamental, especially within the improvement and sending of manufactured insights and prescient analytics, where biases and algorithmic division may incidentally compound health inappropriateness (Gaur et al. 2024).

The fast progression of Meta-Health innovations has outpaced existing legitimate systems and directions, requiring continuous endeavors to adjust and refine arrangements to address developing challenges. Administrative bodies must buildup clear rules for the collection, capacity, and utilization of health information, guaranteeing compliance with laws such as the Healthcare Protections Compactness and Responsibility Act (HIPAA) and the Common Information Assurance Control (GDPR). In addition, systems for risk, negligence, and mental property rights must be upgraded to account for the interesting dangers and obligations related to technology-driven healthcare delivery. Meta-Health advances have the potential to worsen existing societal concerns and well-being aberrations on the off chance that is not carefully executed and observed. It is basic to address value issues related to get to, reasonableness, and social affectability within the plan and arrangement of healthcare advances. Activities to bridge the computerized partition, advance well-being education, and engage marginalized communities within the advancement of technology-driven intercessions are basic for guaranteeing that all people can take advantage of propels in Meta-Health. Moreover, endeavors to moderate algorithmic inclinations, ensure vulnerable populations, and advance comprehensive decision-making forms are basic for cultivating belief and acknowledgement and obtaining Meta-Health innovations.

In other words, exploring the moral, lawful, and social suggestions of Meta-Health innovations requires a multifaceted approach that equates advancement with responsibility, patient-centeredness with protection assurance, and innovative headway with societal value. By maintaining moral standards, adhering to legal systems, and tending to societal concerns, we can guarantee that Meta-Health advances fulfil their guarantee of changing healthcare delivery while defending the rights, nobility, and well-being of all people (Ullah et al. 2023).

As Meta-Health innovations proceed to convert healthcare conveyance, it is basic to address ethical, lawful, and social suggestions (ELSI) to guarantee their dependable and even-handed utilization. Moral contemplations encompassing persistent independence, security, and advantage must direct the improvement and execution of progressed advances. Legitimate systems and controls must be adjusted to address the interesting challenges posed by technology-driven healthcare conveyance, while also protecting understanding rights and guaranteeing responsibility. Besides, endeavors to address societal concerns and value issues are fundamental for cultivating belief, acceptance, and impartiality to Meta-Health innovations. By exploring the complex scene of ELSI, the total potential of Meta-Health innovations to make strides in understanding results, upgrade healthcare conveyance, and advance healthcare value for all has been tackled.

4.4 Integration and Interoperability Challenges

Interoperability in healthcare alludes to the capacity of diverse data frameworks, gadgets, and applications to trade, decipher, and utilize information consistently. Accomplishing interoperability requires the appropriation of standardized information groups, wordings, and communication conventions in healthcare settings. Key interoperability measures incorporate Healthcare Level Seven Universal (HL7),

Quick Healthcare Interoperability Assets (FHIR), and Worldwide Measurable Classification of Maladies and Related Healthcare Issues (ICD). By following interoperability guidelines, healthcare organizations can encourage the consistent trade of healthcare data, progress care coordination, and improve understanding of results. Meta-Health frameworks coordinated different innovations, counting electronic healthcare records (EHRs), telemedicine stages, wearable gadgets, manufactured insights (AI), and genomic information, to provide personalized, data-driven healthcare. Accomplishing consistent integration of these advances requires interoperability at numerous levels, counting information trade, framework compatibility, and workflow integration. By leveraging interoperability measures and opening Application Programming Interfacing (API), healthcare organizations can interface different frameworks and information sources, empowering real-time get to comprehensive persistent data and encouraging collaborative decision-making over care groups. Consistent information trade is fundamental for empowering educated decision-making, personalized healthcare delivery, and effective healthcare operations in Meta-Health frameworks. Be that as it may, accomplishing consistent information trade requires overcoming specialized, organizational, and social boundaries that ruin interoperability. Specialized challenges incorporate information fracture, incongruent frameworks, and information security concerns, which can be tended through information standardization, encryption conventions, and secure information-sharing components. Organizational challenges, such as siloed information stores and competing needs, require collaboration and arrangement among partners to set up information administration structures, motivations, and responsibility instruments. Social challenges, counting resistance to alter and the need for interoperability mindfulness, require instruction, preparation, and social change to cultivate a culture of collaboration, straightforwardness, and shared obligation for interoperability. Integration and interoperability challenges pose significant obstructions to the consistent trade of healthcare data and the realization of Meta-Health systems' full potential. By embracing interoperability benchmarks, joining different innovations, and cultivating culture of collaboration and straightforwardness, healthcare organizations can overcome these challenges and accomplish consistent information trade. Leveraging interoperable Meta-Health frameworks, healthcare suppliers can convey personalized, data-driven care, upgrade persistent results, and move forward the productivity and adequacy of healthcare conveyance (Bang and Kim 2023).

4.5 Case Studies and Real-World Implementations

A few fruitful Meta-Health ventures grandstand the transformative potential of coordination progressed innovations and data-driven approaches into healthcare delivery. For illustration, Venture Songbird, a collaboration between Google and Rising, leverages AI and analytics to make strides results and operational effectiveness (Yonck 2020). Another example is the MyHealthEData initiative by the Centers for Medicare and Medicaid Administrations, which truly speaks for itself in terms of engaging patients in controlling health information and getting individualized healthcare administrations. In addition, programs like the All of Us Research Program and the Precision Medicine Activity further prove the importance of large-scale data collection and analysis for the advancement of personalized medicine and population health (Cohen and Mello 2018).

A few significant lessons learned from successful Meta-Health initiatives include the need to engage with stakeholders, interoperability, and data management. Successful projects place a great deal of emphasis on collaboration among all stakeholders, including patients, healthcare providers, technology developers, and policymakers, such that innovation solutions answer clients' needs and fix real-world challenges. In addition, successful initiatives put a premium on interoperability, for information to be predictably exchanged across systems and platforms in support of the need for informed decision-making and coordination of care. Besides, a robust information management system—including security, security, and consent tools—is another requirement necessary to engender trust, protect participants' rights, and ensure adherence to regulatory requirements. Several factors favor the success or failure of Meta-Health initiatives; some of them are technical complexity, organizational culture, and regulatory mandates.

Effective initiatives generally reap clear goals and defined workflows that back good authority, thus making a venture run with feasible administration and partner arrangement. Successful projects also put great attention to client needs, ease of use, and iterative plan forms; thus the innovation arrangement is friendly and satisfies end-users' prerequisites. Otherwise, ventures may flop because of a requirement for accomplice purchase in, poor or no arranging, or an oversight of consideration to administrative compliance and moral reflections. These can also be specialized challenges, including information split, interoperability issues, and cybersecurity dangers. Case ponders and real-world usage give important bits of knowledge into the victories and disappointments of Meta-Health ventures, advertising profitable lessons for future activities. By looking at fruitful ventures, distinguishing key victory components, and learning from disappointments, healthcare organizations and innovation designers can upgrade their capabilities, relieve dangers, and maximize the effect of Meta-Health arrangements. Moving forward, collaboration, advancement, and patient-centered care will be fundamental for driving the proceeded advancement and selection of Meta-Health advances, eventually moving forward understanding results, improving healthcare conveyance, and forming end of the of healthcare.

4.6 Future Directions and Trends

The long run of healthcare is being molded by a heap of developing advances that hold the potential to revolutionize healthcare conveyance and change understanding results. Artificial intelligence (AI) and machine learning are balanced to play progressively remarkable parts in Meta-Health, empowering predictive analytics, personalized treatment suggestions, and robotized optimal support frameworks. Genomics and accuracy medication will proceed to progress, advertising custom-made mediations based on person hereditary cosmetics and biomarker profiles. Also, telemedicine and farther checking innovations will extend get to care, empowering virtual meetings and farther understanding observing and telehealth intercessions. Other rising innovations, such as blockchain, augmented reality (AR), virtual reality (VR), and nanotechnology, will encourage the capabilities of Meta-Health frameworks, driving innovation and progressing healthcare (Adil et al. 2025).

Looking ahead, long-standing time of healthcare guarantees to be characterized by personalized, preventive, and patient-centered care conveyance models empowered by Meta-Health advances. Predictive analytics and AI-driven experiences will engage healthcare suppliers to expect and address quiet needs proactively, driving to make strides healthcare results and decreased healthcare costs. Additionally, propels in inaccessible checking and telemedicine will empower more open and helpful healthcare administrations, especially for underserved populaces and those living in rustic ranges. Accuracy medication will continue to advance, advertising custom-fitted treatment methodologies that optimize restorative viability and minimize unfavorable impacts, subsequently progressing understanding encounters and quality of life. Furthermore, the integration of computerized healthcare innovations into existence, such as wearable gadgets, versatile healthcare apps, and virtual care stages, will engage people to require control of their healthcare and well-being, advancing preventive behaviors and proactive self-care.

To saddle the complete potential of Meta-Health advances and realize the vision of personalized, data-driven healthcare, partners, and policymakers must collaborate to address key challenges and seize openings. Healthcare organizations ought to prioritize speculations in innovation framework, workforce preparing, and understanding engagement techniques to encourage the selection and integration of Meta-Health arrangements. Additionally, policymakers ought to sanction enactment and administrative systems that advance interoperability, information security, and advancement whereas shielding understanding rights and guaranteeing value of get to healthcare administrations. Additionally, stakeholders across the healthcare biological system, counting suppliers, payers, innovation engineers, analysts, and patients, must work together to set up guidelines, best practices, and rules for the dependable improvement, arrangement, and utilization of Meta-Health advances. By cultivating collaboration, advancement, and a shared vision for long term of healthcare, partners and policymakers can clear the way for a more efficient, effective, and even-handed healthcare framework that enables people, upgrades results, and progresses populace healthcare (Uppamma et al. 2025).

In conclusion, the long run of healthcare is shining with guarantee as developing innovations proceed to change the landscape of healthcare conveyance. By grasping advancement, collaboration, and patient-centered approaches, partners and policymakers can explore the complexities of Meta-Health and shape a future where healthcare is personalized, preventive, and enabling for all.

References

Adil M, Song H, Khan MK, Mastorakis S, Farouk A, Jin Z (2025) Metaverse in health care: security challenges and pathways for future research. IEEE Syst Man Cybernet Mag 11(1):95–106

Baggam DS, Rani S (2025) Metaverse dynamics: transforming healthcare for the future. In: Exploring the metaverse. Academic Press, New York, pp 225–234

Bang J, Kim JY (2023) Metaverse ethics for healthcare using AI technology: challenges and risks. In: International conference on human-computer interaction. Springer Nature Switzerland, Cham, pp 367–378

Chengoden R, Victor N, Huynh-The T, Yenduri G, Jhaveri RH, Alazab M et al (2023) Metaverse for healthcare: a survey on potential applications, challenges and future directions. IEEE Access 11:12765–12795

Cohen IG, Mello MM (2018) HIPAA and protecting health information in the 21st century. JAMA 320(3):231–232

Elabiad S (2025) Navigating the ethical and sustainable frontiers of nanotechnology. SSRN 5079782

Farahat MA, Darwish A, Hassanien AE (2023) The implication of metaverse in the traditional medical environment and healthcare sector: applications and challenges. In: Hassanien AE, Darwish A, Torky M (eds) The future of metaverse in the virtual era and physical world. Studies in big data, vol 123. Springer, Cham. https://doi.org/10.1007/978-3-031-29132-6_7

Gaur L, Gaur D, Afaq A (2024) Ethical considerations in the use of the metaverse for healthcare. In: Metaverse applications for intelligent healthcare. IGI Global, Hershey, pp 248–273

Mazumdar H, Khondakar KR, Das S, Harder A, Kaushik A (2025) Artificial intelligence for personalized nanomedicine; from material selection to patient outcomes. Expert Opin Drug Deliv 22(1):85–108

Mohammed R, Albarrak A (2024) The use of metaverse in the health-care system: a scoping review article. Hail J Health Sci 6(1):24–30

Sujatha R, Sarlinraj M, Mohanraj S, Subash T (2025) Integration of metaverse and AoT into the healthcare system. In: Leveraging metaverse and analytics of things (AoT) in medical systems. Academic Press, New York, pp 15–39

Ullah H, Manickam S, Obaidat M, Laghari SUA, Uddin M (2023) Exploring the potential of metaverse technology in healthcare: Applications, challenges, and future directions. IEEE Access 11:69686–69707

Uppamma P, Padma A, Chithanuru V, Ravula V (2025) Metaverse in healthcare: applications and challenges. In: Exploring the metaverse. Elsevier, Amsterdam, pp 45–68

Wang G, Badal A, Jia X, Maltz JS, Mueller K, Myers KJ et al (2022) Development of metaverse for intelligent healthcare. Nat Mach Intell 4(11):922–929

Yonck R (2020) Heart of the machine: our future in a world of artificial emotional intelligence. Arcade, New York

Chapter 5
Meta-Health Digital Therapeutic Applications

5.1 Introduction

The digital age has brought countless opportunities and transformed many aspects of healthcare and medicine. An interesting focus is digital therapeutics (DTx), which uses cutting-edge technologies such as artificial intelligence, machine learning, and mobile applications to provide patients with personalized and preventive medical care outside of traditional clinical settings. DTx are advanced software applications that assist patients in managing different medical conditions and illnesses. Like medications, DTx products offer scientifically validated outcomes that have a positive impact on a specific condition. This sets DTx apart from other wellness apps and medication reminders, distinguishing it from the competition. The range of disorders and diseases that DTx products cover includes obesity, attention deficit hyperactivity disorder (ADHD), type 2 diabetes, depression, anxiety, congestive heart failure, and numerous others (Radanliev 2024).

The main therapeutic areas based on the different treatment modalities are cognitive behavioral therapy and digital therapies that are useful against the Central Nervous System disorders, which include sleep disorders, depression, anxiety, post-traumatic stress disorder, alcohol and drug addiction, pain relief, and panic disorders. This area is relatively active, with one-third of all development related to DTx. Products for systemic diseases—such as diabetes, cancer, and hypertension—where improvement in lifestyle has a remarkable effect, and diseases where the prognosis management of seriously ill patients is important, apply a lifestyle modification approach. The digital therapies regarding the management of medication use are related to diseases mandating long-term periodic medication use, like asthma, chronic obstructive pulmonary disease, and schizophrenia. Apart from that, digital therapies are developed for amblyopia, the neurological damage caused as an effect of stroke and traumatic injury, and attention-deficit hyperactivity disorder by exploiting neuro-rehabilitation therapy (Armeni et al. 2024).

S. Vyas et al., *Meta-Health*, https://doi.org/10.1007/978-981-96-5844-2_5

5.1.1 Digital Health, Digital Medicine, and Digital Therapeutic

Digital health is the use of a wide array of technologies, platforms, and systems across various sectors of health that facilitate an individual's lifestyle, well-being, and health. Digital health is exemplified by health information technologies, telehealth systems, and clinical care management tools. Digital medicine is a software and hardware product that is evidence-based and used to diagnose and intervene in human health. Remote monitoring devices, digital diagnostics, and digital biomarkers make up digital medicine. One subcategory of digital medicine is digital therapeutics as depicted in Fig. 5.1 (Kim et al. 2024). This is an area where scientifically validated therapeutic interventions occur to prevent, manage, or treat diseases.

Moreover, the recent pandemic of COVID-19 accelerated the integration of digital health technologies, including virtual healthcare systems and data analytics, while different stakeholders strive to adapt to the changing circumstances. The metaverse, in that respect, has turned out to be a very important tool in individual digital therapy as it enables the bridge between healthcare providers and patients to tailor treatments across all fields of healthcare (Hadjiat 2024).

The metaverse, exemplified as a digitized dimension based on virtual reality, provides a unique channel for the delivery of digital therapeutics. It puts patients into simulated environments, allowing for highly personalized and engaging treatment experiences. For instance, people with anxiety disorders can exercise relaxation in the middle of serene virtual landscapes, while those who have phobias can be exposed gradually to things they fear within structured virtual environments. Metaverse enables real-time data collection and analysis, thus empowering health

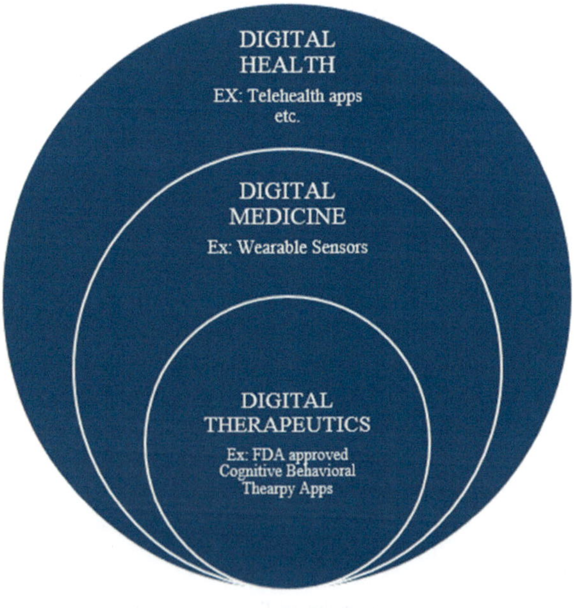

Fig. 5.1 Correlation of digital health, digital medicine, and digital therapeutics

professionals to trace back patients' progress and adjust treatment strategies if needed. It is this breakthrough methodology that can transform mental healthcare, offering treatment alternatives that are accessible, effective, and engaging.

The chapter attempts to provide a comprehensive review on the current impact of metaverse in digital therapeutic interventions, with a specific focus on treatments related to various medical areas.

5.2 The Metaverse and Its Impact on Digital Therapeutics

The metaverse is rapidly transforming the digital world; it greatly influences the digital therapeutics. This union of metaverse technology and healthcare offers a confirming possibility for providing novel and effective therapies (Cho et al. 2024). The introduction of the metaverse into treatment practices can create tectonic changes in the domain of medicine using ordinary technologies. Digital therapeutics (DTx) has taken a prominent position under the healthcare systems, mainly dealing with non-pharmaceutical approaches. Immersive technologies of metaverse such as AR, VR, and XR, alongside Blockchain, AI, and computer vision, are going to provide a new look for telemedicine. With the use of electronic health records (EHRs), digital twins of patients can be designed, permitting 3D simulations for improved healthcare outcomes.

5.2.1 Benefits of Metaverse-Based Digital Therapeutics (DTx)

- **Improved Engagement**: Immersive experiences can contribute to augmented patients' involvement and adherence to treatment.
- **Personalized care**: The metaverse grants designed treatment environments based on patient's needs and preferences.
- **Social Collaboration and Care**: Virtual communities can afford a sense of fit in and support for patients confronting chronic conditions.
- **Data-Driven Perceptions**: Real-time data gathering and analysis can advise treatment decisions and advance outcomes.

5.2.2 Metaverse in Digital Therapeutics (DTx) Areas

- **Mental Health**: Treating situations like depression, anxiety, and PTSD through virtual exposure therapy and cognitive behavioral therapy
- **Chronic Diseases**: Supervising conditions like heart disease, diabetes, and obesity via collaborative games and virtual reality

- **Pain Management**: Delivering distraction methods and recreation tasks in virtual environments
- **Rehabilitation**: Enabling physical therapy and professional therapy in immersive situations

5.3 Prospects of Digital Therapeutics (DTx) in the Meta-Health

The metaverse holds significant potential for revolutionizing digital therapeutics (DTx) by leveraging advanced technologies like AR, VR, XR, blockchain, AI, and computer vision. One of the primary opportunities presented by the integration of DTx and the Meta-Health is the enhanced accessibility to treatment. Virtual worlds offer a convenient and cost-effective platform for individuals to receive therapy, particularly benefiting those who lack access to traditional mental health services, such as individuals residing in rural areas or those who are homebound. DTx in the metaverse enable a high level of personalization. For instance, virtual reality technology can create immersive simulations of specific environments that trigger an individual's anxiety, allowing for targeted treatments that cater to each person's unique needs. Gamification techniques can be employed to make therapy more enjoyable and rewarding, fostering greater participation and adherence. Additionally, the anonymity provided by virtual worlds can facilitate individuals' active engagement in therapy, as they can overcome concerns regarding judgment or social stigma (Lee 2024). There are various DTx opportunities where Meta-Health is the solution:

- **Personalized Treatment**: Therapy environments, highly personalized, could be formulated within the Meta-Health; for example, such treatment could help a patient who has anxiety learn how to relax in an ambient virtual forest or one who has some kind of phobia slowly get desensitized to that fear in a controlled virtual environment.
- **Improved Engagement**: Immersive experiences can also improve the patient's involvement and compliance with treatment. Meta-Health helps in making therapy more interesting which keeps patients motivated and committed to their rehab.
- **Social Collaboration and Care**: Virtual communities are great for fostering belonging and support for people who navigate life with chronic conditions. Members get a chance to interact with others having similar experiences, sharing information, and providing encouragement.
- **Real-Time Data Collection and Analysis**: Meta-Health facilitates the real-time data gathering and processing, which empowers healthcare practitioners to assess patient development and modify treatment strategies as needed. This approach has the potential to enhance care effectiveness and personalization.
- **Remote Accessibility**: Digital therapeutics delivered in the Meta-Health can be accessed from anywhere with an Internet connection, making them more convenient and accessible for patients in remote or underserved areas.

- **Cost-Effective and Scalable Resolutions**: The immersive technologies of Meta-Health can make various therapies extra cost-effective and scalable, permitting for expansive reach and influence in public health projects.

5.4 Use Cases of Digital Therapeutics (DTx) in the Meta-Health

This seamless blend of technology and healthcare in the metaverse is set to revolutionize digital therapeutics, making treatments more effective, accessible, and personalized. Here are some use cases discussed showing the impact of Meta-Health for DTx:

- **Digital Therapeutics (DTx) for Sleep-Wake Disorders and Substance Abuse**: Pear therapeutics has developed a prescription-only DTx application called Somryst for insomnia treatment for above 22 patients. The app works via a method of sleep restriction and consolidation, limiting the time a patient spends in bed to match the amount of time they sleep. It is backed by a clinician-facing dashboard, where healthcare professionals can follow the patients' use of the app, the severity of their symptoms, and their sleep metrics. Pear therapeutics also offers other prescription-only DTx solutions, called reSET and reSET-O, targeting substance use disorders and opioid use disorders via cognitive behavioral therapy, both used in outpatient treatments supervised by clinicians. In the pipeline is reSET-A, a tool designed to target alcohol addiction, which has received Breakthrough Device Designations from the FDA (Orsolini et al. 2024).
- **Atopic Dermatitis (Eczema) Treatment**: Digital therapeutics (DTx) firm Sidekick Health has partnered with pharma giant Pfizer to launch a DTx solution for atopic dermatitis (AD). The collaboration aims to provide a dedicated digital therapeutic solution for the niche area of atopic dermatitis. Patients using the app alongside their regular treatment regime reported a significant reduction in symptoms and improved adherence to treatments and preventive measures.
- **Digital Therapeutics (DTx) Targeting Behavioral Health Conditions**: New York-based Happify offers Ensemble, an app-based exercise program designed to change negative thinking patterns and develop healthy habits. The company has also developed Basis, a nonprescription DTx app for managing symptoms of stress, anxiety, and depression. Both solutions target specific problems and have a well-defined target audience, with Ensemble focusing on changing thinking patterns and Basis addressing symptoms of stress, anxiety, and depression.
- **Cancer Treatment**: Sidekick Health has partnered with Eli Lilly to provide support for Lilly's oncology treatment programs, particularly targeting key pain points in breast cancer treatments. The collaboration will initially launch in Germany, with potential expansion to other countries. The identified pain points in cancer treatment include pain, nausea, anxiety, lack of understanding of the

treatment, and lack of adherence to treatment. Kaiku Health also offers a CE-marked DTx application for various cancer types in multiple countries.

- **Chronic Pain Treatments**: Digital therapeutics (DTx) tools, including virtual reality (VR) therapy, have shown promise in managing chronic pain. Solutions such as RelieVRx and HelloBetter utilize principles of cognitive behavioral therapy to ease chronic pain. AppliedVR, the developer of RelieVRx, is developing applications targeting chronic back pain management, opioid-sparing treatments for various conditions, and pain and anxiety management for specific conditions.
- **Virtual Support Group Therapy**: Patients having similar medical situations can join support groups virtually with the aid of metaverse, in which they can share their experiences, provide shared support, and join in group therapy meetings. Perhaps, this sense of community is most helpful to the patients facing a chronic illness or psychological health challenge.
- **Adaptive Therapy and Real-Time Supervision**: Continuous data collection in the Meta-Health allows real-time monitoring of patient advancement, aiding dynamic variations to treatment plans. This can bring to more receptive therapeutic involvements.
- **Digital Addiction Healing Systems**: Meta-Health can offer immersive programs for addiction recovery, involving virtual meetings, mindfulness methods, and revert inhibition training. These programs can present constant support and a coordinated environment for people in recovery.

These use cases provide a glance into the wide range of open DTx solutions. Each solution focuses on a specific condition or area, addressing well-defined problems and target audiences. The integration of DTx into healthcare and medical practice is an ongoing process, with the potential to empower patients and improve health outcomes.

5.5 Convergence Challenges of Meta-Health and Digital Therapeutics (DTx)

The implementation of DTx for Meta-Health provokes some major challenges (Armeni et al. 2024). These challenges emphasize the requirement of cautious planning, robust setup, and constant research to essentially execute DTx in the Meta-Health (Park 2024):

- **Data Privacy and Security**: Converging digital therapeutics with Meta-Health will engage in sensitive patients information accessing and storing, including health records and real-time biometric data. Privacy and the security of the information are challenging issues as Meta-Health is a highly vulnerable environment. That will protect patient data from hackers, unauthorized use, or breaches which is important for developing trust with regulations including HIPAA and GDPR.

- **Compatibility and Integration**: One of the most significant challenges to achieving DTx in the Meta-Health is integration and compatibility. Multiple virtual worlds run based on their own unique technologies and platforms, so making ones that will work cohesively on most is quite a challenge. Frequent changes in the virtual world will only provoke this problem in maintaining compatibility with digital therapeutics.
- **Stigma and Misconceptions**: Even though treatment for mental health is highly developed in these modern times, it is still subjected to a certain stigma. This could restrict and slow the propagation and acceptance of DTx in the Meta-Health. Moreover, the misunderstandings that DTx are less effective in comparison with traditional therapy are very common, and thus they must be overcome in order that its full potential and recognition about it in terms of efficacy reaches the metaverse.
- **Cost and Funding**: The successful implementation of DTx in the Meta-Health requires substantial resources, involving funding and technical proficiency. There is a potential risk that the cost accompanying with development and delivery of DTx in the Meta-Health may be expensive for some people. Inadequate funding prospects could further hinder access to DTx, mainly for those who stand to benefit the most from these involvements.
- **Regulatory and Ethical Considerations**: The bringing in of DTx into the Meta-Health brings with it a very complicated regulatory and ethical environment. The regulations in health that exist at this time may fail to capture the unique aspects of the virtual reality environments, which creates uncertainty around the approval of Meta-Health-based treatments. Furthermore, ethical affairs about the capability for misuse, the quality of care stipulated, and the digital split must be attended to ensure reasonable access and safe usage of these technologies.

5.6 Potential Advancements in Digital Therapeutics (DTx) for the Meta-Health

The potential for DTx to revolutionize Meta-Health is an exciting prospect, offering numerous advancements and opportunities to enhance patient outcomes and increase access to care (Kwon et al. 2024).

AI-Driven Customized Therapies: The usage of AI in DTx applied within the Meta-Health would most probably allow for extreme personalization in the means of treatment. AI algorithms can evaluate huge amounts of real-time patient data, modifying therapeutic involvements based on individual answers and progress. This level of personalization could lead to more efficient and adapted therapies for situation like mental health disorders, chronic pain, and rehabilitation (Lee 2024).

- **Improved Virtual Reality (VR) and Augmented Reality (AR) Involvements**: As VR and AR technologies revive to evolve, the therapeutic experiences within the Meta-Health could be more immersive and authentic. Better sensory feedback, such as tactual feedback and innovative visualizations, can develop therapeutic exercises and conditions more involving advancing patient loyalty and conclusions. These improvements could be remarkably valuable in areas such as exposure therapy, physical rehabilitation, and cognitive behavioral therapy.
- **Enhancement of Digital Therapeutic Avatars**: Enhanced avatars within the Meta-Health can serve as digital health trainers, counsellors, or friends, presenting personalized supervision and support to patients. These avatars use AI to connect with patients, proposing support, trailing progress, and even providing therapeutic contents. The presence of empathetic and responsive avatars could augment the therapeutic experience, compelling it more significant and participating.
- **Remote Therapeutic Involvements**: The Meta-Health could transform telemedicine by assisting remote therapeutic mediations that are as applicable as in-person treatments. Virtual hospitals and therapy rooms could present secure spaces for patients to accept care from anywhere in the world. This could make high-quality healthcare more available to people in remote areas, decreasing the obstacles to obtaining timely and effective treatment (Park 2024).
- **Cross-Platform Amalgamation and Interoperability**: Developments in cross-platform integration could assist continuous connection between diverse DTx tools and healthcare systems. This would permit patients to move through diverse Meta-Health platforms while sustaining stability in their therapeutic involvements. Increased interoperability would also help better sharing of data and expertise of care beyond distinct healthcare sources.
- **Ethical Framework Development**: As DTx in the Meta-Health advance, there will be requirement for improved regulatory and ethical frameworks that confirm patient data privacy, safety, and the efficacy of therapies. The expansion of these frameworks could help regulate methods, encourage trust among patients, and facilitate the extensive acceptance of Meta-Health DTx (Cho et al. 2024).

5.7 Ongoing Projects Focusing Digital Therapeutics (DTx) in the Meta-Health

Here are some continuing projects and ideas aiming on DTx in the Meta-Health system:

- **XRHealth**: It is utilizing virtual reality (VR) techniques that provide therapeutic training within the Meta-Health systems. Their VRHealth platform proposes various applications for cognitive rehabilitation, where patients can involve in personalized therapeutic encounters within virtual reality. The program is devised to be utilized at home, granting patients to endure therapy remotely with real-time supervising by healthcare workers.

- **MindMaze**: It is a neurotechnology corporation that is establishing DTx solutions in virtual environments. Their program, MindMotion, uses virtual reality to support neurorehabilitation for brain stroke patients. The immersive practices help patients recover mechanical function via involving gamified therapy sessions that can be operated within the Meta-Health.
- **Akili Interactive**: It is emerging DTx video games to treat cognitive conditions. Their leading product, EndeavorRx, has already been accepted by the FDA for the treatment of ADHD in infants. Akili is investigating the assimilation of these therapeutic games into the metaverse, designing virtual environments where patients can contribute in cognitive therapy and training in a more collaborative and immersive mode.
- **BehaVR**: It aims on utilizing VR-based DTx for mental health disorders, such as PTSD, anxiety, and chronic pain. Their platform presents innovative, customized therapy sessions that can be retrieved within the Meta-Health. The corporation is performing on growing its services to involve wider mental health treatments in VR environments.
- **MetaCure**: It is a project targeted at combining DTx into the Meta-Health to direct chronic specifications, for instance, obesity and diabetes. The project invites to generate virtual health training and routine programs that are adapted to patient needs. These programs are devised to participate patients in healthy behaviors via virtual simulations and game-based activities (Lakshmi et al. 2024).
- **BrightBrainer**: It is expanding a metaverse-based platform for cognitive rehabilitation that directs old-age patients with cognitive injuries, like dementia. The platform extends a sequence of interactive, VR-based training and games intended to advance cognitive tasks. Patients can contribute to these activities in the Meta-Health, improving their cognitive skills in a safe and encouraging conditions.
- **Rendever**: It concentrates on reducing social loneliness amid older patients through VR capabilities. Their platform grants seniors to discover virtual worlds, contribute to virtual travel, and participate in group tasks within the Meta-Health. This approach not only improves mental health but also grants therapeutic assistance by supporting social communication and cognitive commitment.
- **VRPhysio**: It is emerging a metaverse-based platform for physiotherapy that permits patients to perform rehabilitation tasks in the virtual world. The platform proposes a variation of exercises that are designed according to patient's requirements and advance in real time. By integrating gamified components, VRPhysio intends to make physical therapy more efficient for patients.

5.8 Conclusion

The integration of digital therapeutics (DTx) into the Meta-Health attends a remarkable opportunity to revolutionize healthcare and improve patient outcomes. By advanced technologies such as artificial intelligence, machine learning, virtual reality, and wearables, DTx offer personalized and accessible solutions for various medical conditions. The potential for DTx in fields like atopic dermatitis, cancer treatment, behavioral health conditions, sleep–wake disorders, and chronic pain management showcases the breadth of possibilities in this emerging field. However, challenges remain in terms of integration and compatibility, addressing stigma and misconceptions, and ensuring affordability and funding for widespread adoption. It is crucial to navigate these challenges to fully unlock the potential of DTx in the metaverse and provide equitable access to quality healthcare. As technology continues to evolve and the metaverse becomes more accessible, there is a significant opportunity to reach underserved populations and provide tailored, effective treatments. The ability to personalize treatment plans using AI and ML algorithms, create immersive environments through VR and AR, and leverage wearables for real-time feedback all contribute to enhancing patient engagement and satisfaction.

The future of DTx in the metaverse holds immense promise. With continued advancements and collaborations between digital health firms, pharmaceutical companies, and healthcare providers, we can anticipate further innovations in mental health treatment, remote healthcare delivery, and improved overall well-being. The seamless integration of DTx into everyday care and medical practice will require ongoing research, investment, and collaboration, but the potential benefits for patient empowerment and better health outcomes make it a compelling endeavor. In conclusion, the combination of DTx and the metaverse has the potential to transform healthcare, providing personalized, accessible, and effective treatments for a wide range of conditions. By leveraging advanced technologies and overcoming challenges, we can create a future where DTx play a vital role in enhancing patient care and well-being in the digital age.

References

Armeni P, Polat I, De Rossi LM, Diaferia L, Meregalli S, Gatti A (2024) Exploring the potential of digital therapeutics: an assessment of progress and promise. Digit Health 10:20552076241277441

Cho CH, Lee HJ, Kim YK (2024) The new emerging treatment choice for major depressive disorders: digital therapeutics. In: Recent advances and challenges in the treatment of major depressive disorder. Springer, Berlin, pp 307–331

Hadjiat Y (2024) Digital health technologies in cancer care and research. Springer, Berlin

Kim M, Patrick K, Nebeker C, Godino J, Stein S, Klasnja P et al (2024) The digital therapeutics real-world evidence framework: an approach for guiding evidence-based digital therapeutics design, development, testing, and monitoring. J Med Internet Res 26:e49208

Kwon H, Choi IY, Kim DJ, Yoo JH (2024) A review of current digital mental health care applications for anxiety symptoms and future prospects. Psychiatry Investig 21(6):551

Lakshmi D, Kondurkar I, Kumar R, Banerjee R (2024) Intelligent healthcare systems in the metaverse: architecture, applications, challenges, and opportunities. In: The metaverse for the healthcare industry. Springer, Berlin, pp 17–32

Lee AG (2024) AI- and XR-powered digital therapeutics (DTx) innovations. In: Digital frontiers-healthcare, education, and society in the metaverse era. IntechOpen, London

Orsolini L, Longo G, Volpe U (2024) Practical application of digital therapeutics in people with mood disorders. Curr Opin Psychiatry 37(1):9–17

Park JY (2024) Current status and future development of digital therapeutics. J Korean Med Assoc/Taehan Uisa Hyophoe Chi 67(2):76–82

Radanliev P (2024) Dance as a mental health therapy in the metaverse: exploring the therapeutic potential of dance movement therapy as a non-pharmacological treatment in the metaverse. Front Comput Sci 6:1334027

Chapter 6
Role of AR/VR/XR/MR in Meta-Health

6.1 Introduction

Augmented reality (AR), virtual reality (VR), extended reality (XR), and mixed reality (MR) are emerging technologies that are reshaping various aspects of healthcare and well-being. This article explores the multifaceted roles of these immersive technologies within the context of "Meta-Health," a holistic approach to well-being that transcends conventional healthcare models (Ficarra 2020). The realm of Meta-Health has seen a transformative impact through the integration of augmented reality (AR), virtual reality (VR), extended reality (XR), and mixed reality (MR) technologies (Ficarra 2020; Kamphuis et al. 2014). These technologies have revolutionized medical diagnostics, treatment, education, and patient experiences. AR allows medical professionals to overlay digital information in the real world, aiding in procedures like surgery by providing real-time data and visual guidance. VR has proven immensely useful for pain management, rehabilitation, and exposure therapy, immersing patients in controlled environments to alleviate discomfort or aid recovery (Kamphuis et al. 2014). Virtual environments provide engaging platforms for rehabilitation exercises, aiding in the recovery process. Additionally, VR has proven effective in stress management and mental well-being, offering therapeutic experiences and relaxation techniques. XR merges physical and virtual realities, enhancing medical training by simulating complex scenarios and offering hands-on experiences in a risk-free environment. MR combines real and digital elements, fostering advanced telemedicine where doctors can remotely visualize and manipulate patient data. From patient education through interactive simulations to assisting surgeons with intricate procedures, these technologies in the realm of Meta-Health have elevated healthcare to new dimensions, providing innovative solutions and improved outcomes (Kamphuis et al. 2014). This article explores the multifaceted roles of these immersive technologies within the context of "Meta-Health," a holistic approach to well-being that transcends conventional healthcare models.

S. Vyas et al., *Meta-Health*, https://doi.org/10.1007/978-981-96-5844-2_6

Moreover, these technologies contribute to data visualization and analysis, enabling medical professionals to comprehend intricate medical data through immersive experiences. As technology continues to advance, the integration of immersive technologies into the Meta-Health paradigm presents new opportunities to enhance healthcare outcomes and empower individuals on their paths to optimal health and vitality.

- **Health Education and Empowerment**: AR, VR, XR, and MR offer interactive and immersive platforms for health education. Through realistic simulations and visualizations, medical professionals can enhance their training, and patients can gain a deeper understanding of their conditions. This empowerment leads to informed decision-making and active participation in personal health management (Silva et al. 2018).
- **Telemedicine and Remote Consultations**: Meta-Health emphasizes the accessibility of healthcare services. AR, VR, XR, and MR facilitate remote consultations and telemedicine by bridging geographical gaps. Patients can connect with healthcare providers virtually, enabling timely interventions and follow-ups, regardless of their location (Barsom et al. 2016).
- **Holistic Mental Health**: Well-being encompasses mental and emotional states. VR provides safe environments for exposure therapy, anxiety management, and meditation. By immersing individuals in calming virtual landscapes, these technologies aid in stress reduction and support mental health treatments (Brigham 2017).
- **Physical Rehabilitation Enhancement**: AR, VR, XR, and MR technologies offer engaging tools for physical rehabilitation. Interactive exercises in virtual environments motivate patients during recovery, enhancing their adherence to rehabilitation routines and ultimately expediting healing (Zhu et al. 2014).
- **Pain Distraction and Management**: Pain perception can be influenced by immersive experiences. VR diverts patients from sensations of pain through medical methods, cutting the need for sedation. Furthermore, chronic pain sufferers can benefit from immersive pain management therapies (Whittemore and Knafl 2005).
- **Surgical Planning and Training**: Surgeons leverage AR, VR, XR, and MR for preoperative planning and training. These technologies enable three-dimensional visualization of patient anatomy, enhancing surgical precision and reducing risks associated with complex procedures (Yoon et al. 2018).
- **Data Visualization and Analysis**: Meta-Health involves understanding complex health data. AR, VR, XR, and MR enable intuitive data visualization, aiding medical professionals in comprehending intricate datasets and making informed decisions (Aggarwal 2010).
- **Lifestyle and Preventive Health**: Immersive technologies can encourage healthy behaviors by making ease of wellness activities. AR, VR, XR, and MR applications promote physical activity, healthy nutrition, and mindfulness, aligning with the preventive focus of Meta-Health (Grant and Booth 2009).

- **Personalized Treatment Approaches**: These technologies enable tailoring interventions to individual needs. By creating personalized simulations and experiences, AR, VR, XR, and MR contribute to treatments aligned with patients' unique contexts (Cook and Reed 2015).
- **Health Monitoring and Feedback**: Meta-Health involves ongoing self-awareness. AR, VR, XR, and MR devices can provide real-time health data visualization, helping individuals monitor their progress and make informed choices (Mewes et al. 2019).

The healthcare sector is embracing innovative concepts, harnessing rapid advancement to significantly benefit human well-being. Predictions indicate a swift expansion in the global execution of AR and VR within healthcare from 2018 to 2025, indicating a transformative influence on the industry (Brigham 2017; Zhu et al. 2014; Whittemore and Knafl 2005). The emergence of technologies like Magic Leap and Microsoft HoloLens in the realm of AR and VR has unlocked novel prospects in healthcare. These immersive visual technologies, jointly mentioned as extended reality (XR), merge virtual and real surroundings. Virtual reality enables complete engagement within a simulated environment, whereas augmented reality overlays virtual components onto the real world, enriching contextual understanding. The integration of AR and VR into healthcare is projected to be a lasting and game-changing element, bolstering safety for both patients and healthcare providers, all while nurturing innovative progress. Mixed reality has a different concept as it depends on the real and virtual environment as shown in Fig. 6.1.

Mixed reality (MR) is a technology that merges components of augmented reality (AR) and virtual reality (VR) to create immersive practices that unite the virtual and physical worlds. In the context of healthcare, MR has several potential applications like medical training, remote consultation, medical imaging, and research and development by visualizing molecular structures and conducting virtual experiments (Kent et al. 2021).

Shown above is the comprehensive analysis of the increased usage of AR (augmented reality), VR (virtual reality), XR (extended reality), and MR (mixed reality) in the healthcare sector that would typically involve a significant amount of data collection, processing, and visualization (Mathew and Pillai 2020). As shown in Fig. 6.2, all the sectors have significantly improved technological interference in the healthcare area for the innovation of the Meta-Health (Yoon et al. 2018). The choice of technology depends on the specific healthcare application. For example, VR may

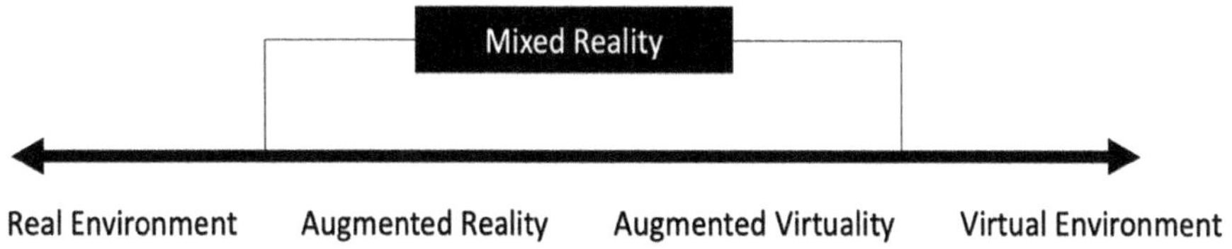

Fig. 6.1 Dimensions in mixed reality (Kent et al. 2021)

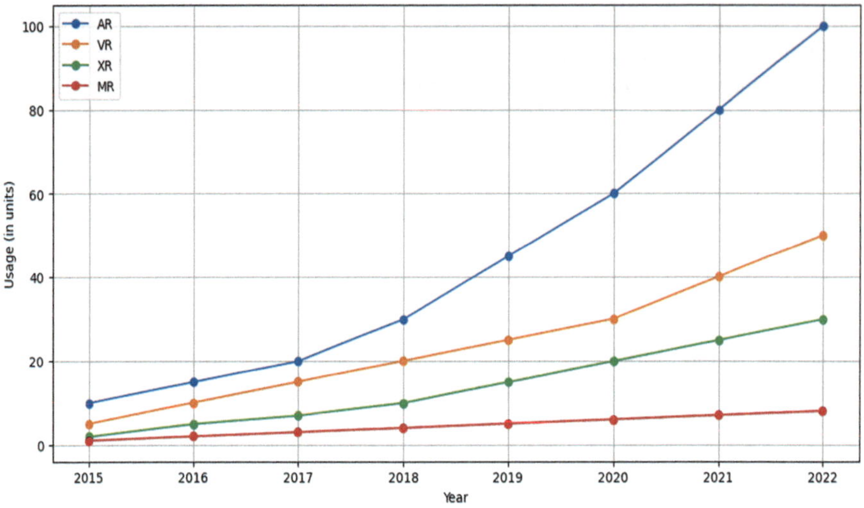

Fig. 6.2 Comprehensive analysis of the increased usage of AR, VR, XR, and MR in healthcare (Mathew and Pillai 2020)

be more prevalent in medical training and rehabilitation, while AR may be more suitable for surgical navigation and remote consultations. XR and MR can bridge the gap amid the virtual and real world and offer more versatile solutions.

Augmented reality (AR), virtual reality (VR), extended reality (XR), and mixed reality (MR) technologies have achieved pivotal importance in the healthcare sector by revolutionizing medical education, patient care, and treatment. AR enhances visualization and surgical precision, facilitating complex surgeries, while VR aids in medical training and pain management. XR offers versatile applications, connecting real and virtual worlds for diverse healthcare needs, and MR advances medical imaging, diagnostics, and treatment planning. These immersive technologies not only improve healthcare training, enhance patient understanding, and enable remote consultations but also embrace the potential to upsurge the accurateness and competence of medical measures, eventually leading to improved patient outcomes and advancing the healthcare industry into a more technologically driven future (Whittemore and Knafl 2005; Yoon et al. 2018; Aggarwal 2010).

6.2 Augmented Reality (AR) and Healthcare

Augmented reality (AR) in healthcare is a rapidly evolving field that holds significant promise for transforming medical research and clinical practice (Gerup et al. 2020). This chapter will provide a thorough assessment of the applications and implications of AR in healthcare, offering valuable insights into its role as a revolutionary technology for research within the healthcare sector. AR is transforming the healthcare industry by effortlessly merging digital information and virtual components with the real world (Gerup et al. 2020; Ferrari et al. 2019). It enhances medical training, surgery, and patient care in numerous ways, enabling medical professionals to visualize complex anatomical structures, practice procedures, and access real-time patient data through AR headsets or mobile devices. Patients can benefit from AR applications for remote consultations, personalized treatment plans, and improved understanding of their conditions (Jha et al. 2021). This immersive technology holds immense potential to optimize healthcare delivery, reduce errors, and enhance the overall patient experience by bringing cutting-edge digital tools into the hands of medical practitioners and their patients (Jha et al. 2021).

6.2.1 Application of AR in Medical Education and Training

In the area of medical training and education, AR has appeared as a transformative tool. It permits aspiring healthcare practitioners to engage in immersive, hands-on learning experiences. Students can use AR applications to explore detailed 3D models of anatomical structures, visualize disease progression, and practice surgical procedures in a risk-free virtual environment. Moreover, AR enhances medical simulations, enabling trainees to gain valuable experience and refine their skills. It also facilitates real-time collaboration among students and instructors, bridging geographical gaps for remote learning (Viglialoro et al. 2021). As a result, AR not only improves the quality of medical education but also contributes to more confident and competent healthcare professionals, ultimately enhancing patient care and safety (Viglialoro et al. 2021).

6.2.2 Surgical Navigation and Visualization

Augmented reality (AR) is rapidly advancing surgical navigation and visualization in the healthcare industry. Surgeons can now access real-time, highly detailed, 3D interpretations of the patient's anatomy through AR headsets or smart glasses during procedures. This technology allows for precise and personalized surgical planning, aiding in the navigation of complex anatomical structures with greater accuracy. Surgeons can superimpose digital overlays of critical information, such as preoperative scans, instrument locations, or even augmented guidance pathways, onto the patient's body in real time (Moro et al. 2017). This enhances the surgeon's situational awareness, reduces the risk of errors, and leads to more minimally invasive and efficient surgeries. In addition, AR assists in remote collaboration, enabling expert consultation from anywhere in the world. Surgical navigation and visualization through AR not only improve surgical outcomes but also pave the way for new frontiers in telemedicine and global healthcare access (Viglialoro et al. 2021; Moro et al. 2017).

6.2.3 Diagnostic Support and Imaging

AR is playing significant role in diagnostic support and medical imaging by providing healthcare professionals with innovative tools to enhance their diagnostic accuracy and decision-making. AR systems can overlay crucial patient data, like lab test report data, medical images, and real-time patient vitals, directly onto the clinician's field of view. This real-time information integration helps doctors to better understand a patient's condition and make more informed diagnoses. In radiology, AR can assist in visualizing and interpreting complex imaging studies, offering 3D reconstructions and highlighting specific areas of interest, thereby improving diagnostic precision. Furthermore, AR-based diagnostic support systems can guide practitioners in performing medical procedures with unparalleled accuracy (Ma et al. 2014). By combining real-world and digital information seamlessly, AR is transforming the way medical professionals analyze data, finally indicating to quicker and more precise diagnoses and, subsequently, more effective patient care.

6.2.4 Remote Consultations and Telementoring

Augmented reality (AR) is participating a pivotal role in remote healthcare delivery, mainly in the realms of remote consultations and telementoring. AR technology enables healthcare providers to conduct virtual consultations with patients, leveraging real-time video streams and digital overlays to share medical information, discuss treatment plans, and offer guidance. Moreover, AR facilitates telementoring by allowing experienced medical experts to remotely assist and mentor less experienced colleagues during surgeries or procedures. This interactive and immersive experience bridges geographical distances, enhances the quality of care, and fosters knowledge transfer in real time (Ma et al. 2014; Bui et al. 2021). As a result, AR is breaking down barriers to access to specialized healthcare expertise, remarkably in remote or underserved areas, while maintaining high standards of medical practice and education. It is a critical enabler of telemedicine and telementoring, improving healthcare access and outcomes for patients across the globe (Ma et al. 2014).

As shown in the pie chart in Fig. 6.3, it visually represents the proportion of AR usage in healthcare for each of the specified years. The highlighted slice for 2023 emphasizes the increasing trend, showing that AR usage is expected to reach 60% by that year. This chart provides a clear and concise way to convey the growth of AR technology adoption in the healthcare sector over the 5-year period (Ara et al. 2021; Cheng et al. 2016; Jensen and Konradsen 2018). The estimated market size for augmented in the healthcare sector worldwide was approximately $2.4 billion in 2022, with a projected growth to reach about $14.07 billion by 2032. This growth corresponds to a compound annual growth rate (CAGR) of 19.4% projected in the forecast period from 2023 to 2032 (Ara et al. 2021; Jensen and Konradsen 2018).

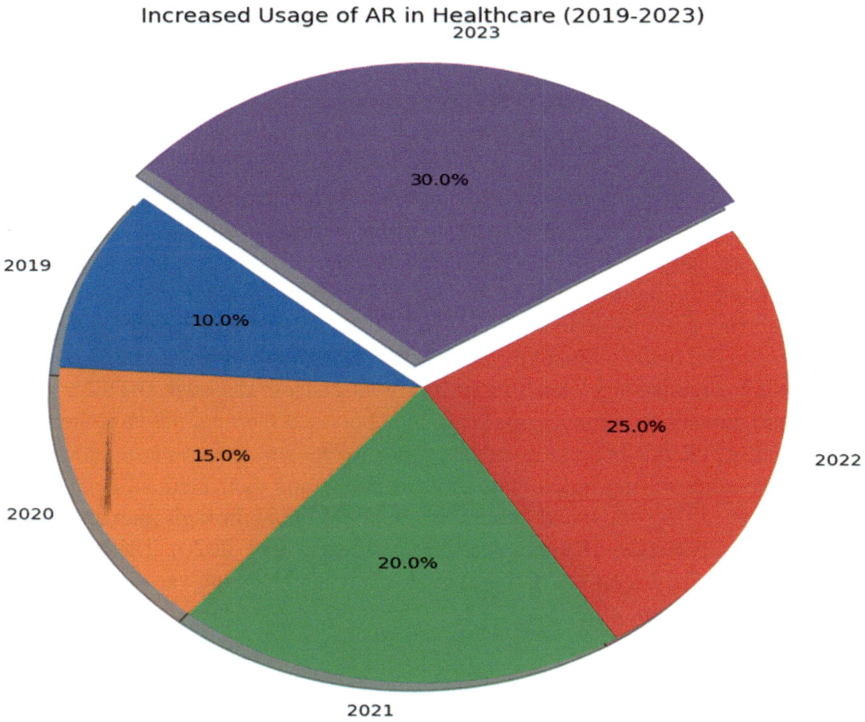

Fig. 6.3 Augmented reality usage in healthcare (Ara et al. 2021)

6.3 Virtual Reality (VR) and Healthcare

Virtual reality (VR) is a transformative technology with significant applications in the healthcare sector, providing a dynamic and immersive environment that has the potential to transform numerous aspects of healthcare, from medical teaching and treatment to patient care and diagnostics. In this chapter, it is essential to delve into the specific aspects and implications of VR in healthcare (Dermody et al. 2020). VR is a technique that has transcended the boundaries of the gaming and entertainment industry, making significant inroads into the field of healthcare. VR, with its immersive and interactive capabilities, has opened a realm of possibilities which were once contemplated as a science fiction. In the context of healthcare, VR offers a dynamic platform for patient care, medical training, therapy, and research, thereby transforming the way we approach various aspects of the healthcare ecosystem (Dermody et al. 2020; Saab et al. 2022).

6.3.1 Application of VR in Healthcare

Applications of virtual reality (VR) in healthcare are diverse and promising. VR technology has emerged as a powerful tool for medical education and training, presenting immersive environments for students and specialists to practice surgical techniques, investigate anatomical structures, and enhance diagnostic skills (Saab et al. 2022). It is also extensively used for surgical planning and simulation, enabling surgeons to rehearse complicated procedures with accuracy and safety. Beyond the operating room, VR plays a key role in pain management and rehabilitation, offering patients nonpharmacological alternatives for pain relief and therapeutic exercises. In the realm of psychological therapy and wellness, VR is utilized for treating circumstances such as posttraumatic stress disorder (PTSD), paranoias, and anxiety by engaging patients in supervised therapeutic environments. Additionally, VR has become a valuable tool for patient engagement and health promotion, empowering individuals to well understand their medical conditions, make informed decisions, and adhere to treatment plans through interactive and educational experiences (Saab et al. 2022; Triegaardt et al. 2020). These applications showcase the versatility and potential of VR in enhancing various aspects of healthcare (Triegaardt et al. 2020).

6.3.2 Benefits of Virtual Reality (VR) in Healthcare

The advantages of VR in healthcare are multifaceted and transformative. VR enhances medical training by presenting immersive simulations for trainee physicians, increasing their skills and belief while minimizing the risks correlated with traditional hands-on training. In the realm of surgery, VR aids in preoperative planning, offering precise, patient-specific models for surgeons to practice on, finally leading to enhanced surgical accuracy and patient safety (Saab et al. 2022). Moreover, VR is proving to be an effective tool for nonpharmacological pain management, offering distraction and relaxation techniques that alleviate pain and reduce the need for pain medications. In psychological therapy and wellness, VR offers a safe and moderate environment for experience therapy and stress reduction. Additionally, the immersive nature of VR fosters higher patient commitment and devotion to treatment regimens, promoting better health outcomes (Triegaardt et al. 2020). These collective advantages underscore VR's potential to significantly enhance the quality of healthcare and patient experiences.

6.3.3 Future Outlooks of Virtual Reality in Healthcare

The future of healthcare promises to be dynamic and transformative, with several key prospects and trends shaping the landscape. One prominent trend is the continued integration of telemedicine and telehealth services, offering improved access to medical care and consultations, particularly in remote and underserved areas. AI plays a fundamental role in improving diagnostic accuracy, predictive analytics, and personalized treatment plans (Fertleman et al. 2018). Wearable health tech, including smartwatches and fitness trackers, will further encourage individuals to observe and supervise their health proactively. The advent of 5G technology will revolutionize data transmission and connectivity, facilitating real-time patient monitoring and telemedicine (Laver 2020). Moreover, healthcare systems are increasingly focusing on preventive and holistic approaches, emphasizing wellness and mental health, as well as addressing social determinants of health to create a more inclusive and equitable healthcare ecosystem. These trends, among others, are poised to redefine the future of healthcare, making it more patient-centric, efficient, and technologically advanced (Laver 2020; Mallik et al. 2022; Javaid et al. 2022) (Table 6.1).

Table 6.1 Applications of virtual reality in healthcare (Mallik et al. 2022; Javaid et al. 2022)

Application	Description
Medical training	VR is used for training medical professionals, offering realistic simulations for surgical procedures, anatomy exploration, and patient diagnosis
Pain management	VR diverts patients from pain through medical techniques or chronic pain management by immersing them in soothing virtual environments
Physical rehabilitation	VR-based exercises and activities assist in physical therapy and rehabilitation for patients recovering from injuries or surgeries
Exposure therapy	VR exposes patients to phobias, PTSD (posttraumatic stress disorder) triggers, or anxiety-inducing conditions in a monitored and safe environment to facilitate with therapy and desensitization
Cognitive rehabilitation	VR assists patients with cognitive impairments or neurodegenerative conditions in memory training and mental exercises
Surgical planning	Surgeons use VR to plan complex surgeries, practicing and visualizing the procedure before operating on a patient
Psychological therapy	VR is used in psychological therapy for treating various mental health conditions such as depression, anxiety, and PTSD (posttraumatic stress disorder)
Wellness and relaxation	VR provides wellness programs, meditation sessions, and relaxation experiences for stress reduction and mental health improvement

6.4 Mixed Reality (MR) and Healthcare

Mixed reality (MR) in healthcare is a pioneering technology that seamlessly blends the physical and virtual worlds to revolutionize patient care, medical training, and research. By overlaying holographic digital content, like 3D medical scans or patient data, onto the real world, MR empowers healthcare professionals to visualize and interrelate with complex medical information in real time (John and Wickramasinghe 2020). Surgeons can perform surgeries with augmented guidance, medical students can practice on virtual patients, and clinicians can better understand patient data. Additionally, MR enhances telemedicine by enabling remote specialists to collaborate in shared mixed reality environments. This technology progresses patient outcomes and accelerates medical education and advances the overall quality of healthcare delivery (John and Wickramasinghe 2020; Stretton et al. 2018). The benefits of MR in Meta-Health are discussed as follows:

- **Real-Time Diagnostic**: Real-time diagnostics in mixed reality (MR) represent an advanced technology in healthcare. By integrating augmented virtual information into the physical clinical environment, MR enables healthcare professionals to access real-time diagnostic data and imaging directly during patient examinations. For instance, during surgery, surgeons can view 3D medical images superimposed on the patient's body, aiding in precise navigation and better decision-making (Stretton et al. 2018). MR facilitates instant access to patient records, diagnostic imaging, and real-time monitoring, streamlining the diagnostic process and permitting for more precise and efficient decision-making. This innovation could substantially improve patient care by reducing errors, increasing diagnostic speed, and enhancing the overall quality of healthcare diagnostics and treatment (Stretton et al. 2018).
- **Improved Medical Training**: Mixed reality (MR) is transforming medical training in healthcare by presenting a dynamic and immersive learning experience. Medical students and professionals can now engage with lifelike 3D anatomical models and patient scenarios, linking theory and practice (Ficarra 2020). MR simulations allow for realistic surgical training, enabling trainees to practice methods constantly and upgrade their skills in a riskless environment. This technology also supports collaborative learning, as students and instructors can interact with virtual patients and medical scenarios together, despite of physical location. By combining real-world experience with the advantages of virtual environments, MR is revolutionizing medical education, ultimately producing better prepared and more competent healthcare practitioners, improving patient safety, and driving advancements in the field (Martin et al. 2020).
- **Image-Guided Surgery**: Image-guided surgery using mixed reality (MR) in healthcare is a transformative approach that combines the precision of medical imaging with the immersive capabilities of MR technology to enhance surgical procedures. Surgeons wear MR headsets that overlay real time, 3D images, such

as CT scans and MRI reports, onto the patient's anatomy during surgery. This enables surgeons to see vital structures, like blood vessels or tumors, that may not be visible to the naked eye (Martin et al. 2020; Stantchev 2010). As they operate, they can receive immediate feedback and guidance, allowing for more accurate, minimally invasive procedures. MR can also assist in preoperative planning, making it easier to locate incision points and avoid critical areas. This technology improves surgical accuracy, reduces difficulties, reduces recovery times, and finally improves patient results. It represents a meaningful advancement in the field of surgery and is becoming increasingly prevalent in various healthcare specialities (Stantchev 2010).

As shown with the above represented data in Fig. 6.4, since 2017 the usage of mixed reality (MR) in healthcare has experienced a significant surge, with the technology making substantial strides by 2023. Healthcare professionals have increasingly adopted MR applications to augment medical training, clinical planning, and patient care. Physicians now use MR-based simulations to refine their skills and practice complex procedures, reducing the risk of errors in real surgeries. Additionally, MR has revolutionized medical education, offering immersive learning experiences for students and enabling remote training for healthcare workers (Fu et al. 2022). Furthermore, MR-assisted diagnostics and telemedicine have allowed for more accurate and remote patient assessments, improving accessibility to healthcare services. Overall, the integration of MR technology with Meta-Health has transformed the healthcare landscape, advancing innovative solutions and improved patient outcomes (Fu et al. 2022; Hu et al. 2019b).

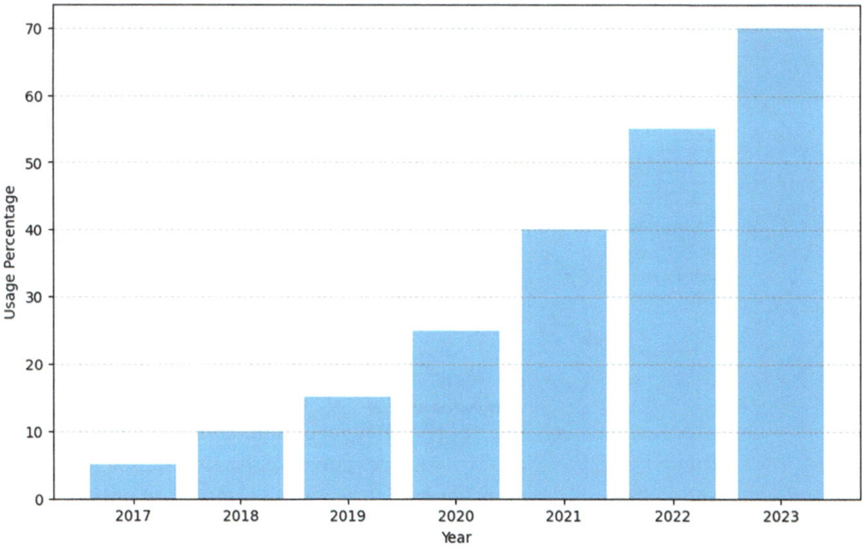

Fig. 6.4 Increased usage of mixed reality in healthcare (Hu et al. 2019a; Kobayashi et al. 2018)

6.5 Extended Reality (XR) in Healthcare

Extended reality (XR), which incorporates augmented reality (AR), virtual reality (VR), and mixed reality (MR), holds immense importance in healthcare. This technology has revolutionized the medical field by presenting innovative resolutions that enhance medical training, diagnostics, medication, and patient care (Logeswaran et al. 2021). XR applications allow healthcare specialists to simulate complex procedures, improving their skills and reducing errors in surgery. Moreover, XR enables more accurate and efficient patient assessments, remote consultations, and even immersive therapeutic interventions. With XR, healthcare is becoming more accessible, efficient, and patient-centric, making it a pivotal tool in the advancement of modern healthcare practices (Logeswaran et al. 2021; Kerdvibulvech and Dong 2021).

As shown in Fig. 6.5, extended reality (XR), a cooperative term encircling virtual reality (VR), augmented reality (AR), and mixed reality (MR), plays an essential role in transforming healthcare practices in numerous ways. All the potential application of the XR depends upon the elements of AR/VR/MR which are explained as follows:

- **Medical Training and Education**: XR technology offers a dynamic platform for medical scholars and experts to obtain hands-on experience and enhance their

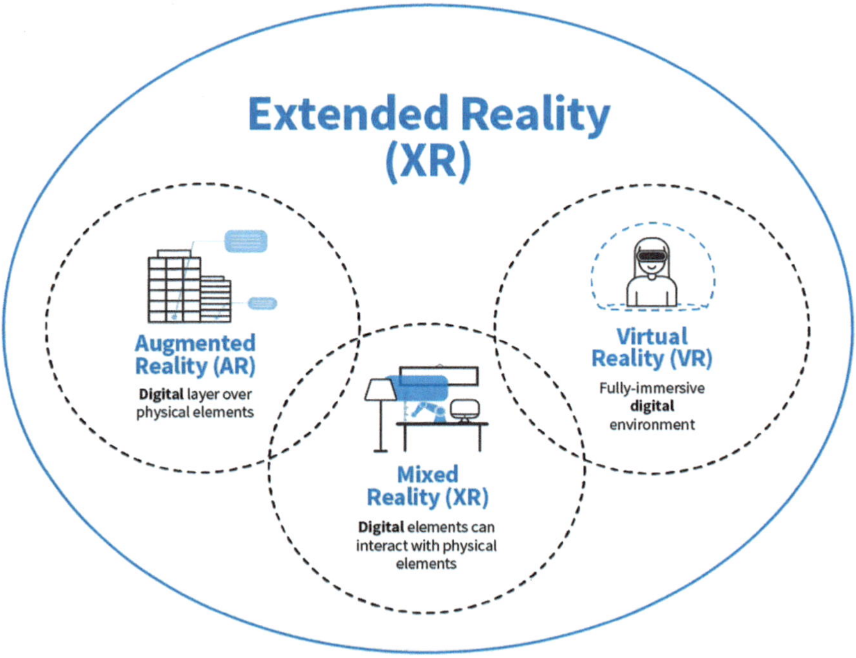

Fig. 6.5 Integration of AR/MR and VR for XR

skills. VR-based simulations provide a safe and supervised environment for practicing surgical procedures, allowing trainees to make errors and understand from them without risking patient safety. This immersive learning experience is invaluable for honing surgical skills and improving the overall quality of healthcare professionals (Kerdvibulvech and Dong 2021).

- **Telemedicine and Remote Consultations**: XR technologies are making telemedicine more effective. Patients can receive remote consultations with specialists who can use AR to examine medical records or MR to visualize and explain complex medical conditions in a way that is easy for patients to understand. This expands approach to healthcare services, specifically for those in remote areas (Shaikh et al. 2023).
- **Patient Education and Engagement**: XR can also serve as a powerful tool for patient training and engagement. Patients can utilize AR applications to better understand their medical situation, treatment options, and postoperative care. This augments patient compliance and encourages individuals to take an effective role in handling their health (Vyas 2023).
- **Data Visualization and Analytics**: XR can be used to visualize dense medical data, allowing healthcare professionals to gain deeper insights into patient conditions and treatment outcomes. This helps in making more informed decisions and personalized treatment plans (Andrews et al. 2019).
- **Accessibility and Inclusivity**: XR technologies are making healthcare more accessible and inclusive. Patients with mobility issues, incapacities, or controlled access to healthcare facilities can gain from XR-powered telemedicine and remote monitoring, reducing disparities in healthcare access (Andrews et al. 2019).

The importance of extended reality in healthcare lies in its ability to improve medical training, enhance surgical procedures, broaden access to healthcare services, and engage patients in their own care. As XR maintains to develop its applications in healthcare will likely grow, extending even more innovative and efficient solutions to improve patient outcomes and the overall healthcare experience (Vyas 2023; Andrews et al. 2019).

As shown in Fig. 6.6, the increased usage of extended reality (XR) in various healthcare sectors has catalyzed a transformative wave in the industry. In medical training and education, XR has become indispensable, offering immersive, risk-free environments for students and professionals to refine their skills and practice complex procedures. Surgical planning and visualization have also seen remarkable advances, with XR applications providing real-time guidance for precise surgeries, reducing risks and enhancing patient outcomes (Pons et al. 2022). Telemedicine has been revolutionized, making remote consultations more effective and accessible, while XR-assisted diagnostics are providing deeper insights and more accurate assessments. Patient engagement has improved with XR-driven therapies and educational tools, authorizing persons to take control of their health. As XR endures to evolve, its applications in healthcare, from pain management to data analytics, promise to reshape the future of medicine, enhancing patient care and reducing healthcare variations (López-Ojeda and Hurley 2021).

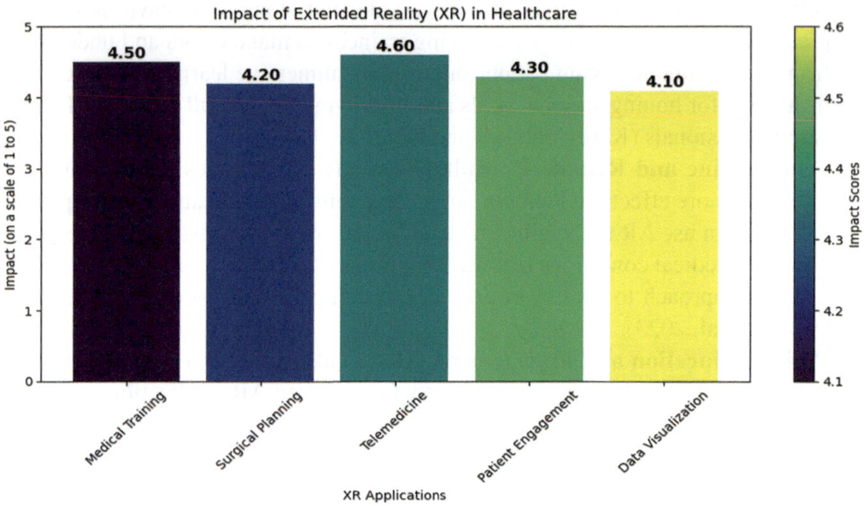

Fig. 6.6 Showing increased usage of extended reality in different areas of healthcare (Pons et al. 2022)

6.5.1 Use Cases of XR in Improvising Healthcare Systems

The integration of XR in healthcare is unveiling fresh prospects for healthcare professionals and presents an advantageous horizon, particularly for contemporary healthcare. XR technologies offer the potential to support surgeons within the operating room, streamlining the process of accessing critical information for time-sensitive decisions. Key applications of XR in the healthcare realm encompass the training of emerging medical practitioners and delivering patients a more profound comprehension of diseases or ailments (López-Ojeda and Hurley 2021; Zhang et al. 2023).

The above use cases as shown in Table 6.2 highlights how XR technologies are employed in both Meta-Health and traditional healthcare to enhance well-being, educate and engage patients, and support medical professionals in their daily practices (Takemoto et al. 2020).

Extended reality (XR) is proving to be a versatile tool with numerous use cases in both Meta-Health (wellness and well-being) and traditional healthcare. In the realm of Meta-Health, XR applications provide immersive wellness and fitness experiences, offering users gamified physical exercises, meditation environments, and personalized dietary advice (Kundi 2022). These technologies also enable the monitoring of physical activities, vital signs, and nutritional intake. They foster engagement and education, motivating individuals to adopt healthier lifestyles. In the healthcare sector, XR plays a pivotal role in medical teaching, granting students and healthcare experts to practice surgical procedures in a safe, virtual environment (Innocente et al. 2022). It aids in mental health therapy, utilizing exposure therapy

Table 6.2 Some significant use cases of the XR in improvising the healthcare system (Takemoto et al. 2020)

Use case	Meta-Health	Medical and healthcare
Mental health therapy	XR can provide therapeutic environments for stress reduction, anxiety management, and meditation	XR-based therapies are used for exposure therapy in treating conditions such as PTSD and phobias
Health and fitness tracking	XR devices can track physical activities and offer real-time data on steps taken, heart rate, and more	XR is used to monitor patients' vital signs and offer real-time data to medical staff for better patient care
Diet and nutrition support	XR apps can provide personalized dietary advice, track nutritional intake, and assist in meal planning	XR applications can visualize nutritional information for patients, aiding them in making healthier dietary choices
Telehealth and remote consultations	XR can facilitate virtual wellness sessions and consultations with wellness coaches and nutritionists	XR technology enables remote consultations with healthcare professionals, especially in telemedicine scenarios
Data visualization and analysis	XR devices can display personal wellness data and trends for users to monitor and adjust their health goals	XR can visualize complex medical data for analysis, aiding in diagnostics, treatment planning, and research

for conditions like PTSD, and physical rehabilitation post-injury or surgery. XR enhances telehealth by enabling remote consultations and patient monitoring, while also contributing to pain management and data visualization for medical analysis. In both domains, XR is revolutionizing how we approach well-being and healthcare, offering innovative solutions to improve patient outcomes and overall health and wellness (Ahmad et al. 2023; Gasteiger et al. 2022).

6.6 Conclusion

First and foremost, the integration of AR and VR is expected to become more seamless and sophisticated. This study focuses on the empowerment of healthcare professionals to have instantaneous access to patient information, medical records, and real-time data during procedures, significantly improving decision-making and the overall quality of care. Moreover, the applications of VR are likely to extend beyond surgical training to immersive therapeutic interventions, allowing patients to manage pain, and anxiety, and even undergo cognitive behavioral therapies in a virtual world.

In the realm of MR and XR, we anticipate more widespread use in surgical settings. The ability to overlap digital information on top of the real-world surgical environment offers unmatched precision and guidance, reducing the margin for error in complex procedures. This advancement could lead to smaller recovery times and progressed patient results. The role of these immersive technologies in

Meta-Health is undeniably transformative. These immersive technologies have already demonstrated their significance in medical training, surgical planning, patient engagement, and telemedicine. The significance of AR and VR lies in their ability to provide lifelike simulations and enhanced learning experiences for medical professionals, while MR and XR offer real-time, data-rich insights into patient conditions. As these technologies continue to advance, the future perspective is exceptionally promising. They have the potential to transform how Meta-Health is delivered, making it more available, efficient, and patient-centric. From improving diagnostics and treatment planning to enhancing remote consultations and rehabilitation, AR, VR, MR, and XR are set to contribute significantly to the advancement of Meta-Health. They hold the key to reducing disparities in healthcare access and empowering both healthcare professionals and patients to make well-versed decisions.

The data visualization and analytics capabilities of AR, VR, MR, and XR are likely to revolutionize research and diagnostics. These technologies will enable healthcare professionals to process complex medical data swiftly, facilitating early disease detection and specified treatment strategies. Likewise, the integration of AI and ML with XR will offer predictive analytics, improving preventive care and early intervention. As we move forward, it is crucial to address ethical and privacy terms in the employment of these technologies and ensure that they remain accessible and equitable for all, reducing healthcare disparities. With these considerations in mind, the future holds immense potential for AR, VR, MR, and XR to advance healthcare to unprecedented heights, ultimately improving patient outcomes, quality of care, and the overall human experience in the healthcare domain.

References

Aggarwal A (2010) The evolving relationship between surgery and medicine. AMA J Ethics 12(2):119–123

Ahmad HF, Rafique W, Rasool RU, Alhumam A, Anwar Z, Qadir J (2023) Leveraging 6G, extended reality, and IoT big data analytics for healthcare: a review. Comput Sci Rev 48:100558

Andrews C, Southworth MK, Silva JN, Silva JR (2019) Extended reality in medical practice. Curr Treat Options Cardiovasc Med 21:1–12

Ara J, Karim FB, Alsubaie MSA, Bhuiyan YA, Bhuiyan MI, Bhyan SB, Bhuiyan H (2021) Comprehensive analysis of augmented reality technology in modern healthcare system. Int J Adv Comput Sci Appl 12(6):840–849

Barsom EZ, Graafland M, Schijven MP (2016) Systematic review on the effectiveness of augmented reality applications in medical training. Surg Endosc 30:4174–4183

Brigham TJ (2017) Reality check: basics of augmented, virtual, and mixed reality. Med Ref Serv Q 36(2):171–178

Bui DT, Barnett T, Hoang HT, Chinthammit W (2021) Tele-mentoring using augmented reality technology in healthcare: a systematic review. Australas J Educ Technol 37(4):68–88

Cheng A, Kessler D, Mackinnon R (2016) Reporting guidelines for health care simulation research: extensions to the CONSORT and STROBE statements. Adv Simul 1:25

Cook DA, Reed DA (2015) Appraising the quality of medical education research methods: the medical education research study quality instrument and the Newcastle–Ottawa scale-education. Acad Med 90(8):1067–1076

Dermody G, Whitehead L, Wilson G, Glass C (2020) The role of virtual reality in improving health outcomes for community-dwelling older adults: systematic review. J Med Internet Res 22(6):e17331
Ferrari V, Klinker G, Cutolo F (2019) Augmented reality in healthcare. J Healthc Eng 2019:9321535
Fertleman C, Aubugeau-Williams P, Sher C, Lim AN, Lumley S, Delacroix S, Pan X (2018) A discussion of virtual reality as a new tool for training healthcare professionals. Front Public Health 6:44
Ficarra B (2020) Virtual reality, augmented reality, and mixed reality. In: Emerging technologies for nurses: implications for practice. Springer, New York, pp 95–126
Fu Y, Hu Y, Sundstedt V (2022) A systematic literature review of virtual, augmented, and mixed reality game applications in healthcare. ACM Trans Comput Healthc (HEALTH) 3(2):1–27
Gasteiger N, van der Veer SN, Wilson P, Dowding D (2022) Exploring how, for whom and in which contexts extended reality training 'works' in upskilling healthcare workers: a realist review. In: 2022 IEEE conference on virtual reality and 3D user interfaces abstracts and workshops (VRW). IEEE, Piscataway, pp 734–735
Gerup J, Soerensen CB, Dieckmann P (2020) Augmented reality and mixed reality for healthcare education beyond surgery: an integrative review. Int J Med Educ 11:1
Grant MJ, Booth A (2009) A typology of reviews: an analysis of 14 review types and associated methodologies. Health Inform Librar J 26(2):91–108
Hu HZ, Feng XB, Shao ZW, Xie M, Xu S, Wu XH, Ye ZW (2019a) Application and prospect of mixed reality technology in medical field. Curr Med Sci 39:1–6
Hu H, Shao Z, Ye L, Jin H (2019b) Application of mixed reality technology in surgery. Int J Clin Exp Med 12(4):3107–3133
Innocente C, Ulrich L, Moos S, Vezzetti E (2022) Augmented reality: mapping methods and tools for enhancing the human role in healthcare HMI. Appl Sci 12(9):4295
Javaid M, Haleem A, Singh RP, Khan S (2022) Understanding roles of virtual reality in radiology. Internet Things Cyber-Phys Syst 2:91–98
Jensen L, Konradsen F (2018) A review of the use of virtual reality head-mounted displays in education and training. Educ Inf Technol 23:1515–1529
Jha G, Sharma LS, Gupta S (2021) Future of augmented reality in healthcare department. In: Proceedings of second international conference on computing, communications, and cyber-security: IC4S 2020. Springer Singapore, Singapore, pp 667–678
John B, Wickramasinghe N (2020) A review of mixed reality in health care. In: Delivering superior health and wellness management with IoT and analytics. Springer, Berlin, pp 375–382
Kamphuis C, Barsom E, Schijven M, Christoph N (2014) Augmented reality in medical education? Perspect Med Educ 3:300–311
Kent L, Snider C, Gopsill J, Hicks B (2021) Mixed reality in design prototyping: a systematic review. Des Stud 77:101046
Kerdvibulvech C, Dong ZY (2021) Roles of artificial intelligence and extended reality development in the post-COVID-19 era. In: HCI international 2021-late breaking papers: multimodality, eXtended reality, and artificial intelligence: 23rd HCI international conference, HCII 2021, virtual event, July 24–29, 2021, proceedings 23. Springer International Publishing, Berlin, pp 445–454
Kobayashi L, Zhang XC, Collins SA, Karim N, Merck DL (2018) Exploratory application of augmented reality/mixed reality devices for acute care procedure training. Western J Emerg Med 19(1):158
Kundi GM (2022) Virtual reality in healthcare: exploring the patients' behavior through the lens of extended stimulus, organism, and response framework. Open Access Public Health Health Admin Rev 1(1):9–25
Laver K (2020) Virtual reality for stroke rehabilitation. In: Virtual reality in health and rehabilitation. CRC Press, Boca Raton, pp 19–28
Logeswaran A, Munsch C, Chong YJ, Ralph N, McCrossnan J (2021) The role of extended reality technology in healthcare education: towards a learner-centred approach. Future Healthc J 8(1):e79

López-Ojeda W, Hurley RA (2021) Extended-reality technologies: an overview of emerging applications in medical education and clinical care. J Neuropsychiatry Clin Neurosci 33(3):A4-177
Ma M, Jain LC, Anderson P (eds) (2014) Virtual, augmented reality and serious games for healthcare 1, vol 1. Springer, Berlin
Mallik R, Patel M, Atkinson B, Kar P (2022) Exploring the role of virtual reality to support clinical diabetes training—a pilot study. J Diabetes Sci Technol 16(4):844–851
Martin G, Koizia L, Kooner A, Cafferkey J, Ross C, Purkayastha S et al (2020) Use of the HoloLens2 mixed reality headset for protecting health care workers during the COVID-19 pandemic: prospective, observational evaluation. J Med Internet Res 22(8):e21486
Mathew PS, Pillai AS (2020) Role of immersive (XR) technologies in improving healthcare competencies: a review. In: Virtual and augmented reality in education, art, and museums. IGI Global, Hershey, pp 23–46
Mewes A, Heinrich F, Kägebein U, Hensen B, Wacker F, Hansen C (2019) Projector-based augmented reality system for interventional visualization inside MRI scanners. Int J Med Robot Comput Assist Surg 15(1):e1950
Moro C, Štromberga Z, Raikos A, Stirling A (2017) The effectiveness of virtual and augmented reality in health sciences and medical anatomy. Anat Sci Educ 10(6):549–559
Pons P, Navas-Medrano S, Soler-Dominguez JL (2022) Extended reality for mental health: current trends and future challenges. Front Comput Sci 4:1034307
Saab MM, Landers M, Murphy D, O'Mahony B, Cooke E, O'Driscoll M, Hegarty J (2022) Nursing students' views of using virtual reality in healthcare: a qualitative study. J Clin Nurs 31(9–10):1228–1242
Shaikh TA, Dar TR, Sofi S (2023) Evolution and contribution of extended reality in smart healthcare systems: toward a data-centric intelligent healthcare approach. In: Extended reality for healthcare systems. Academic Press, New York, pp 159–208
Silva JN, Southworth M, Raptis C, Silva J (2018) Emerging applications of virtual reality in cardiovascular medicine. JACC Basic Transl Sci 3(3):420–430
Stantchev V (2010) Enhancing health-care services with mixed reality systems. In: The engineering of mixed reality systems. Springer, Berlin, pp 337–356
Stretton T, Cochrane T, Narayan V (2018) Exploring mobile mixed reality in healthcare higher education: a systematic review. Res Learn Technol 26:2131
Takemoto JK, Bratelli RA, Parmentier BL, Merritt TA, Coyne L (2020) Extended reality in patient care and pharmacy practice: a viewpoint. J Contemp Pharm Pract 66(4):33–38
Triegaardt J, Han TS, Sada C, Sharma S, Sharma P (2020) The role of virtual reality on outcomes in rehabilitation of Parkinson's disease: meta-analysis and systematic review in 1031 participants. Neurol Sci 41:529–536
Viglialoro RM, Condino S, Turini G, Carbone M, Ferrari V, Gesi M (2021) Augmented reality, mixed reality, and hybrid approach in healthcare simulation: a systematic review. Appl Sci 11(5):2338
Vyas S (2023) Extended reality and edge AI for healthcare 4.0: systematic study. In: Extended reality for healthcare systems. Academic Press, New York, pp 229–240
Whittemore R, Knafl K (2005) The integrative review: updated methodology. J Adv Nurs 52(5):546–553
Yoon JW, Chen RE, Kim EJ, Akinduro OO, Kerezoudis P, Han PK et al (2018) Augmented reality for the surgeon: systematic review. Int J Med Robot Comput Assist Surg 14(4):e1914
Zhang J, Lu V, Khanduja V (2023) The impact of extended reality on surgery: a scoping review. Int Orthop 47(3):611–621
Zhu E, Hadadgar A, Masiello I, Zary N (2014) Augmented reality in healthcare education: an integrative review. PeerJ 2:e469

Chapter 7
Meta-Health Data Privacy and Security

7.1 Introduction to Meta-Health Data Privacy and Security

Meta-Health is a revolutionary intersection of healthcare times big data and digital technologies. Therefore, it is a deep repository that gathers health data from different sources such as, but not limited to EHRs, wearable devices, social media, and genomics. So promising it is the huge possibilities that this data ecosystem creates in transforming healthcare delivery through personalized medicine, predictive analytics, and improved patient outcomes. Whereas the integration of huge volumes of sensitive health data does provide unparalleled opportunities, this dramatically raises a host of challenges—particularly with regard to data privacy and security. The digitization of health has increasingly brought forth concerns regarding the protection of patient information. With increased connectivity among the Meta-Health systems, sharing data between sources becomes more frequent and thereby calls for assuring their safety against unauthorized access and misuse of patient information. Besides the violation of confidentiality, the integrity and reliability of health systems are also compromised by risks that arise from breaches in data privacy and security. The multifaceted nature of privacy concerns in Meta-Health touches on specific debates: ownership of data, consent by patients, and how to balance access to data with strong privacy protections. Finally, healthcare providers and organizations should follow a tough landscape of regulations touching on privacy, such as the HIPAA in the USA and the General Data Protection Regulation in Europe, which impose strict requirements on how personal health information must be handled (https://www.meta-health.info/privacy-policy/).

Since it is an extremely valuable and sensitive information, on the security front, Meta-Health data is inarguably the premier target of cyber threats. With the increase in sophisticated varieties of cyberattack targeting the healthcare sector, among them are ransomware, phishing attacks, and insider threats, which can lead to a data breach. This may have quite serious consequences; hence, encryption, access control, and continuous monitoring are very critical steps toward protection against

S. Vyas et al., *Meta-Health*, https://doi.org/10.1007/978-981-96-5844-2_7

threats and maintaining the resiliency of the Meta-Health systems. The current chapter discussed the most critical aspects of Meta-Health data in terms of privacy and security, with reference to main challenges and regulatory frameworks that should be adopted by any healthcare organization in its effort to secure patient information. We aim to provide an overall review of evolving Meta-Health and of strategies to be required for addressing related security and privacy issues to support health data safely and efficiently in the digital era.

7.2 Definition and Scope of Meta-Health

The Meta-Health paradigm is an emergent healthcare approach, associated with deep integration of health-related data from EHRs, wearable devices, genomics, medical imaging, and social media, among other digital sources. The concept of Meta-Health involves more than just traditional health data; instead, it seeks to address a wide spectrum of information that can be assessed for a holistic view regarding the health status and behavior of a particular individual. It lets actionable insight into generation through advanced analytics, machine learning, and AI, thus allowing personalized medicine, predictive healthcare, and much-informed decision-making by providers of healthcare. The Meta-Health addresses ways in which big data may be leveraged to improve patient outcomes, advance the Prevention Care, and innovate the efficiency of healthcare systems. On the other hand, the huge and interconnected nature of Meta-Health data raises many challenges, in particular, about data privacy and security and governance. Thus, large volume, speed, and variety require robust mechanisms for data management; hence, strict conformation to standards of privacy and security to protect sensitive health information from data breach and misuse accordingly requires being in place. Furthermore, Meta-Health involves complex navigations on ethical and regulatory grounds, insofar as the entirety of reality involves not only patient-specific data but also aggregated information with implications for public health policies and research. Consequently, the definition of Meta-Health and its scope are continuously evolving, shifting with technology development and an ongoing process of juggling between the aspiration to sort out the privacy and security issues with a view to maximizing the benefits for healthcare innovation (https://www.cyrixhealthcare.com/meta-health-a-modern-approach-in-healthcare.php).

7.2.1 Importance and Impact on Healthcare

It is a paradigm shift in data collection, its analysis, and, importantly, how it would be used to improve care and outcomes for patients. The impact of Meta-Health on healthcare would be immense, as it will bring all kinds of data together, such as those from EHRs, wearables, mobile health applications, and even social media, in a united approach toward healthcare. This will give a much bigger view of the patient's health by the healthcare professional, including lifestyle and genetic data and physiological findings in real time, which will lead to more accurate diagnoses and treatments. Applying advanced analytics and AI to this treasure trove, Meta-Health enables predictive modeling for early interventions that can sharply lower chronic disease incidence, improve patient management, and enhance strategies of preventive care. The impact of Meta-Health also extends to healthcare organizations themselves, where analytics-driven decisions can lead to the best use of resources, reduction in the wastage of time and resources, and thereby a reduction in operational costs. For instance, predictive analytics will estimate patient admissions to optimize bed management and plan in advance the resources to be made available. This will help achieve greater efficiency in providing health services. Moreover, Meta-Health is important to progress research and innovation by ensuring that large volumes of various datasets speed up the discovery of new treatments, the development of personalized medicine, and comprehension of population health trends.

However, Meta-Health has some drawbacks; integrating such a vast amount of sensitive health data raises a number of concerns about data privacy, security, and ethics. Trust in digital health solutions can only be achieved by ensuring confidentiality and integrity of patient information. In sum, successful implementation of Meta-Health will only be possible with a proper framework of data governance, complete compliance with regulatory standards, and the development of secure technologies to avoid breaches and other forms of cyber threats. This, together with the challenges, underlines the potential Meta-Health has to change healthcare for the better: improving patient outcomes, enhancing efficiency, and driving innovation-standpoints that will constitute foundational elements in the future of healthcare (https://www.metabase.com/learn/grow-your-data-skills/data-fundamentals/data-types-overview).

7.3 Overview of Data Types in Meta-Health

By summary, Meta-Health brings together under one umbrella a wide array of data types, each one complementing others to give a full overview of the person's health condition, behavior, and environment. This includes a wide range of data types integrated from different sources in order to enable better decision-making for healthcare providers and researchers and personalized delivery. Major types of data in Meta-Health include the following:

1. EHRs are the electronic form of a medical history for a patient, which includes diagnoses, medications, treatment plans, dates of immunization, allergies, radiology images, and other laboratory test results. EHRs make up the foundation of Meta-Health—a digital, clinical, structured platform that fundamentally establishes the basis for patients' care and continuity.

2. Wearable and IoT Devices: Wearable devices, such as fitness trackers and smartwatches, generate streams of real-time data on vital signs, physical activities, and sleep patterns, among other health-related metrics. IoT devices in healthcare also add to the kind of data that includes connected glucose monitors or smart inhalers for continuous monitoring and management of chronic conditions.
3. Omics and Biomarker Data: Genomic data involves DNA sequence data that carry genetic markers of disease, targeted treatment by the patient's own genomic profile; biomarker data is made up of proteins, genes, or other molecular markers, which assist in the early detection of a disease as well as in monitoring the effective results of treatment.
4. Medical Imaging Data: X-ray, MRI, CT, and ultrasound are examples of medical imaging tests that provide valuable visual information regarding the internal structure of the patient. Advanced image analysis techniques using AI-driven interpretations could improve diagnosis and help in precision medicine.
5. Patient-generated health data refers to data that originates with the patient directly, including symptoms, lifestyle, and diet, among other factors, and self-reported outcomes through mobile health applications, patient portals, or surveys. PGHD is really powerful in the valued insight it provides into daily life in a patient and can really inform more personalized care strategies.
6. Social Determinants of Health (SDOH): SDOH data represents the conditions with which people live, work, and play: socioeconomic status, educational background, employment status, and access to healthcare services. It is very pertinent to addressing health disparities and making interventions that take into account the greater context of a patient's life.
7. Pharmacological Information: The knowledge regarding the medication use, including prescription, compliance, side effects, and interactions, plays a cardinal role in the management of the treatments of patients and in the prevention of adverse drug events. It can be used in the optimization of pharmacotherapy and to support programs of medication management.
8. Behavioral and Mental Health Information: This involves data on diagnosis of psychiatric disorders, behaviors, levels of stress, and psychological tests. The approach in integrating behavioral health information into physical health information offers comprehensive patient care.
9. Environmental Data: It is the sum of everything that can influence the health of a person, including the air quality, the rate of pollution, whether it be sunny or rainy, and where one lives. The integration of this environmental data aids in the assessment of risk along with developing prevention concerning people.
10. Administrative and Financial Data: It deals with the consumption of care, billing information regarding patients, claims, and the overall cost incurred. This would be quite useful for analysis in improving healthcare delivery to make it cost-effective and patient-satisfactory.

These sources, coming from a wide array of data types, stand at the center of Meta-Health as it propagates health insight and improvement in a multidimensional way. The integration and analysis of these sources further facilitate the movement toward more predictive, preventive, and personalized healthcare in driving innovation in improved patient outcomes along every point in the continuum of care.

7.4 Meta-Health Data Privacy

Such data includes sensitive health information, ranging from conventional clinical data to personal, behavioral, and genomic data from a variety of digital sources. The protection of Meta-Health data is an important issue in this setting. The huge integration of data coming from EHRs, wearable devices, and patient-generated inputs is raising colossal challenges in terms of privacy because all these datasets may disclose very substantial information on the health of a person, his habits, or even genetic predisposition. Data privacy in Meta-Health is based on strict conditions of privacy principles and standards set by HIPAA in the USA and by the GDPR in Europe, outlining how personal health information is collected, stored, and shared. Key privacy measures include the use of data anonymization and de-identification techniques to protect patient identities while enabling research and analysis to make use of such data. Consent by the patients and ownership of such data are paramount: individuals must have explicit control over who accesses their health data and for what purpose. With more artificial intelligence and machine learning taking hold, requiring large datasets and inadvertently eliciting the re-identification of anonymized data, these concerns regarding privacy are growing. It is a balance between enabling access to data in facilitating healthcare innovations while ensuring the protection of patient privacy—a challenge not that easy to achieve. Healthcare organizations, therefore, have a strong reason to implement substantial data governance frameworks, encryption methods, and access controls to protect the data from breach incidents and unauthorized access. These are crucial topics that have to be overcome in the further development of Meta-Health if the goal is to sustain patients' trust and ensure benefits from integrated health data without compromising individual privacy.

7.4.1 Privacy in Meta-Health

In Meta-Health, privacy is complex and originates with the collection and sharing of large volumes of sensitive health information from multiple sources, such as EHRs, wearable devices, genetic data, and patient-reported outcomes. One of the major issues with such systems is unauthorized access and data breaches, which lead to exposure of sensitive personal health information that may further cause identity theft, discrimination, or other possible misuses by malicious actors. Cyber threats are considered one of the most serious risks facing Meta-Health because of the interconnectedness of these systems, which expands the attack surface. It goes without saying that this does make robust data security measures both highly necessary and challenging to implement across all platforms consistently (Watters 2023). Re-identification of anonymized data is another critical issue. Even for data that is de-identified, advanced analytics might cross-refer with other datasets to sometimes reveal the individual identities, at the risk of patient confidentiality. The use of AI and machine learning in Meta-Health raises issues around algorithmic bias and ethical use of patient data, as it is reliant on large datasets for collection and analysis. This is compounded by the difficulty in informed consent on the part of the patient, as data is usually passively gathered through devices, or it is aggregated from multiple sources, which bars any single individual from truly understanding or controlling how their data may be put to use. The global nature of Meta-Health data sharing also provides challenges regarding disparate laws and regulations with respect to privacy across borders. This adds complexity to compliance and data governance. These concerns for privacy underline the need for sound frameworks regarding privacy, active management of data by the patients themselves, and transparently clear policies that would secure the advancement of Meta-Health without compromising individual rights to privacy.

7.4.2 Main Privacy Principles and Standards (For Example, HIPAA, GDPR)

At the heart of any privacy principles and standards are the Health Insurance Portability and Accountability Act (HIPAA) and General Data Protection Regulation (GDPR), which have set requirements and provided a foundation for keeping health data private and secure within Meta-Health. These two have stipulated the standards that a healthcare organization—and even a data processor—should take for ensuring the triad of confidentiality, integrity, and availability of personal health information.

- Health Insurance Portability and Accountability Act (HIPAA): This is a federal regulation in the USA that establishes the standards to protect health information. The Privacy Rule forms a crucial base for setting safeguards in the protection of the privacy of individually identifiable health information; the Security Rule identifies those standards designated to ensure electronic health information is protected and the standards related to the Breach Notification Rule, which requires notification to individuals of breaches concerning their unsecured protected health information. Thus, the emphasis of HIPAA is on patient consent, minimum necessity, and the right to have access to their own health information. In that respect, the organization is required under HIPAA to adopt the adequate administrative, physical, and technical measures to prevent unauthorized access or improper disclosure of health data.

- GDPR: General Data Protection Regulation is a sweeping data protection regulation applied in the European Union and is applicable to all organizations processing personal data of individuals within the EU, including Meta-Health data. Key principles of GDPR reflect lawfulness, fairness, and transparency in data processing; purpose limitation, which means data processing should be done for specifically stated, explicit, and legitimate purposes; data minimization, ensuring only data that is relevant is processed; accuracy, needing data to be up to date; storage limitation, which dictates that data should be retained only as long as necessary; requirements for the integrity and confidentiality of data; and accountability, requiring organizations to prove that they are compliant with the requirements of the GDPR. The GDPR also gives individuals some important rights: the right to access one's data, the right to rectify, the right to delete (also known as the right to be forgotten), and the right to data portability.
- Other privacy standards besides HIPAA and GDPR, there are other frameworks of privacy standards that are of immense applicability in Meta-Health. For instance, ISO/IEC 27701 is an internationally adopted standard that details the requirements and provides guidance for establishing, implementing, maintaining, and improvement of a Privacy Information Management System. Additionally, other major regulations that impact data privacy with Meta-Health are PIPEDA in Canada and the California Consumer Privacy Act within the USA.

Together, these principles and standards create a resilient foundation that will aid in the protection of Meta-Health data, while guiding organizations through the ethical and legal handling of sensitive health information. The enforcements of these frameworks do more than protect patient privacy; they boost trust and confidence in digital health solutions, knowing that data is being managed responsibly and securely.

7.4.3 Data Anonymization and De-identification Techniques

Data anonymization and de-identification still stand out as some of the major techniques in Meta-Health that aim to offer protection to patient privacy with polices calling for the permissibility to date use of health data in research, analysis, and other secondary uses. The techniques involve alteration or removal of personal identifiers from health data to prevent identification traces of individuals, hence reducing the possibility of breach of privacy.

- Data Anonymization: The process of anonymization is applied to irreversibly transform data so that information identifying a target can no longer directly or indirectly be linked to a person. The objective is to render the risk of re-identification, even by linking the data with other sets of data, negligible. The general methods of anonymization involve generalization, in which specific data will be replaced by their more general descriptions, such as exact ages or precise locations changing to age ranges or city-level locations. The other way is suppression of certain data fields. Another methodology involves randomization, whereby the changes in data values nullify the linkage to the entity while retaining much of the data utility, an example being the addition of noise to numerical values. Properly anonymized data does not fall under certain regulatory requirements such as the GDPR or the HIPAA, respectively, as it ceases to be personal data.

- Data De-identification: De-identification is a weaker form of data transformation than anonymization; the latter decreases the risk of identification rather than fully eliminating it. This would include methods for deletion or generalizing the specific identification of such things as names, addresses, social security numbers, or another direct identifier. Unmasking methods include Masking, a process of modifying data values (e.g., substitution of names by pseudonyms), and Tokenization, a process whereby sensitive data elements are replaced by their corresponding nonsensitive equivalents known as tokens, which are, under the specific conditions described in this document, persistent and of no further use in revealing the original state. According to the HIPAA Privacy Rule, de-identification has two standards: the Expert Determination standard, through which an expert legitimately concludes that the identity risk is quite minimal, and the Safe Harbor standard, which involves exclusion of 18 types of identifiers from the data.
- Challenges and Considerations De-identification and anonymization are important to secure the privacy of patients, but they contain their share of challenges. The following methods are subject to two key concerns: the risk of re-identification through linking the anonymized or ide-identified dataset with other datasets to uncover personal identity, particularly in cases with big datasets or sophisticated data analytics. At times, the following techniques lower the utility of the collected data, such that it becomes unusable for both research and clinical decision-making objectives. The selection of anonymization or de-identification techniques should be judiciously made, keeping in perspective the use case intended on the basis of prevalent regulatory requirements. A good governance framework, continuous monitoring, and technical measures like those of differential privacy will further solidify these methods of Meta-Health data protection. These methods form part of the holistic approach toward data privacy, where healthcare organizations balance risks to individual privacy with the value from health data (Abouelmehdi et al. 2018).

7.4.4 Patient Consent and Data Ownership

These are the twin pillars: patient consent and ownership of data. Without them, the privacy and ethical use of health data do not stand in Meta-Health. With a growing trend in the integration and use of more and more health data, it equally becomes of paramount importance to ensure that the patient has control over their personal information to foster trust and compliance with legal and ethical standards.

- Patient Consent: The second principle deals with consent from the patient, which is an informed permission. It is among the critical needs in healthcare data management. Examples of Meta-Health consent include clarity and understanding of intended use, storage, and sharing with patients. It includes but is not limited to data types; collection purposes, such as treatment or research activities and analytics; and third-party access. As the RM should be done, consent to collect or process personal data should be obtained upfront and must be ongoing as well. It must be a persistent process that allows the patient to review and update his/her consent preferences at any time. Consenting for data handling in clinical medicine is one of the mainstays of ethical stamping, and regulations like the GDPR require that any consent has to be explicit, informed, and freely given. This secures that the patient is enabled to be completely informed and thus consents to data usage rights for protection of autonomy and privacy.
- Data Ownership: This term means the rights and control of persons upon their individual health-related information. In Meta-Health, the notion of ownership representation is inclusive of patient access, control, and full management of health information. It must include rights over access to one's own health record and the right to rectify inaccuracies and to demand the erasure of data. Each patient should have an active role in taking part in the decision of who should use the data and for what: clinical care, research, or marketing. It would include the right to withdraw consent and to have data removed in case that people no longer wish to take part in data-sharing activities. Data ownership has a close affinity with the principles of data protection and privacy; it puts one in a position of ownership in safeguarding his or her information and seeing to it that data is put to use in ways agreeable and expected by an individual.

One could say that effective consent by patients and data ownership practices might be difficult to implement in Meta-Health given the complexity of the ecosystems where data would be managed, or different legal requirements across various jurisdictions. One of the most critical challenges will be to make the processes of consent not only legally compliant but also user-friendly—where the patient is given options clearly and gets easy access to information about his or her data. This would also involve data ownership rights in the case of aggregated and secondary use data, which are harder to manage in terms of ensuring transparency and control. These also include issues of data portability, where ease should be accorded in the transferring of data to other care providers or platforms upon a patient's request. These are the issues that need to be taken cared of: there is a significant demand for consent management systems within healthcare organizations, besides transparent data policies and mechanisms through which patients would be able to realize their rights. In this way, patients would be involved in managing their data, and their preferences may be taken into account. The aim of such measures is to instill trust in the use of Meta-Health data and ensure ethical practices.

7.4.5 Challenges in Balancing Data Sharing and Privacy

Balancing Data Sharing and Privacy: This challenge involves striking a balance between the wide use of data and the protection of individual privacy, which is not easy to achieve in Meta-Health. Figure 7.1 shows the different challenges for the balancing data and privacy. Challenges that will be served as main obstacles for this balance include the following:

1. Data Security and Risk of Breaches: Ensuring that wide data sharing does not become a synonym for increased vulnerability to data breaches and cyberattacks is still one of the main challenges. Accordingly, sharing health data across a host of platforms, organizations, and systems increases the vulnerability toward unauthorized access, theft of data, and malicious activities. Application of strong security measures like encryption, access control, and periodic security audits among others becomes a must. However, such measures can be quite elaborate and expensive.
2. Risks of Anonymization and Re-identification: While anonymization and de-identification methods provide a reasonable level of protection for privacy, they are not fail-safe. Advanced analytics, coupled with access to more auxiliary data, may reidentify certain individuals even from anonymized datasets. The trade-off between the utility of shared data and the efficiency of anonymization is an open challenge that could only be resolved through sophisticated techniques and vigilance.

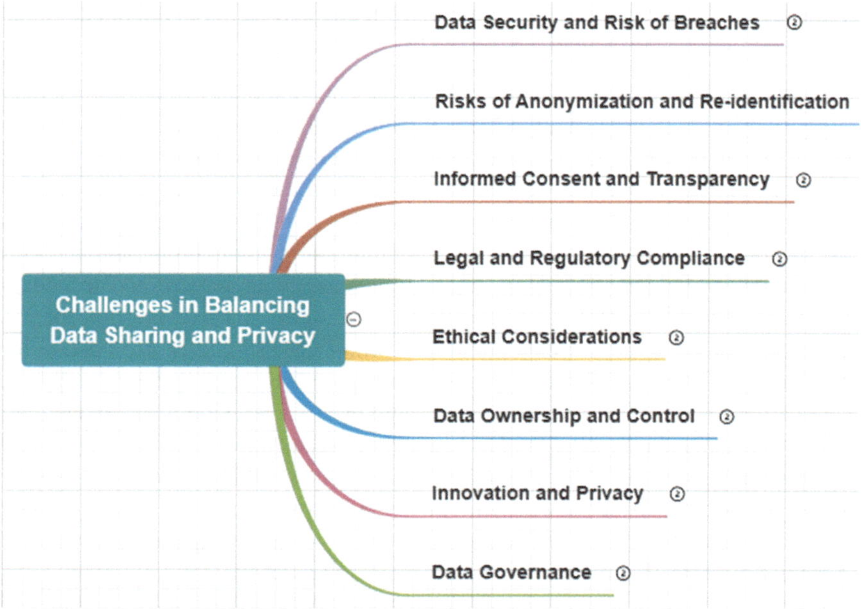

Fig. 7.1 Challenges in balancing data sharing and privacy

3. Informed Consent and Transparency: One big challenge is the explicit consent process and making the patients understand how and where their data is to be used. Events where the sharing of data is well-thought-out, including any possible secondary use for research or commercial events. Transparency in terms of data practices is very much essential; however, acquiring it is indeed a challenging task in complex data ecosystems where multiple stakeholders get involved.
4. Legal and Regulatory Compliance: The increasingly diverse and dynamic environment of data privacy regulations, such as GDPR, HIPAA, and other various regional laws, further complicates this issue. Varied data protection requirements, consent, and breach notification in different jurisdictions put organizations to the test when borders are crossed. Harmonizing data sharing practices with regulatory requirements needs in-depth planning and continuous adaptation.
5. Ethical Considerations: The balance between data sharing and privacy itself is surrounded by a host of ethical issues. When health data is misused for purposes other than what the patient could reasonably have foreseen or consented to, it would mean erosion of trust in the healthcare system. Making certain that data is used responsibly and ethically while facilitating research and innovation serves as one of the challenging key issues in data management.
6. Data Ownership and Control: Ownership of health data by one or more entities and determination of who has control of health data in various shared and collaborative environments is complex. The patient may feel a loss of control about his or her own data as that data is shared across entities. Ensuring meaningful patient control and choice is crucial but clearly hard to effectively implement.
7. A Delicate Balance between Innovation and Privacy: On the one hand, data sharing may be accelerating innovation, improving service delivery in health, and promoting research. On the other side of the scale, unhampered data sharing has been seen as threatening to tear down privacy and security. It takes reflective policy-making and technological solutions that find that right balance in favor of innovation at the same time it protects privacy.
8. Data Governance: Adequate data governance is required to manage the scale and trade-offs between data sharing and privacy. It is about defining policies, protocols, and roles with regard to handling, access, and sharing of data; however, elaborating and managing such a governance framework is quite resource- and time-consuming and complex.

Such challenges require a multifaceted approach, ranging from proper data protection to transparent consent, regulatory compliance, and ethical use of the data. All these factors need to be balanced properly against each other to maximize benefits from data sharing for healthcare organizations while maintaining privacy and public trust.

7.5 Security of Health Data in Meta-Health

Meta-Health-data security means integration of a variety of data sources and advanced technologies. Therefore, critical attention needs to be given to the protection of sensitive health information. The integral parts of good data security are strong encryption of data, both during transmission and at rest; strict access using role-based authentication and multifactor controls; and techniques for masking sensitive information while analyzing it. That finds the vulnerabilities for compliance through continuous monitoring and periodic security audits. The lifecycle of health data is taken cared of through appropriate data storage and proper deletion practices. Along with maintaining regulations like HIPAA and GDPR, detailed training to employees is necessary, along with a clearly identified incident response plan, which plays a great role in the integrity of data and for avoiding breaches with unauthorized access. The application of these measures will help to keep the Meta-Health data secure, which otherwise would not be utilized effectively in patient care and research along with maintaining privacy and compliance standards.

7.5.1 Security Threats in Meta-Health Data

Security threats in Meta-Health data range from vulnerabilities that pose a precarious effect on sensitive health information as shown in Fig. 7.2 in terms of confidentiality, integrity, and availability. These include the following:

1. Cyberattacks and Data Breaches: There is a possibility of cyberattacks with ransomware, phishing, or malware against the systems of Meta-Health in order to gain illicit access or encrypt sensitive health data. The data breaches caused by such attacks may be very serious in terms of loss of patient information, financial costs, and erosion of trust.

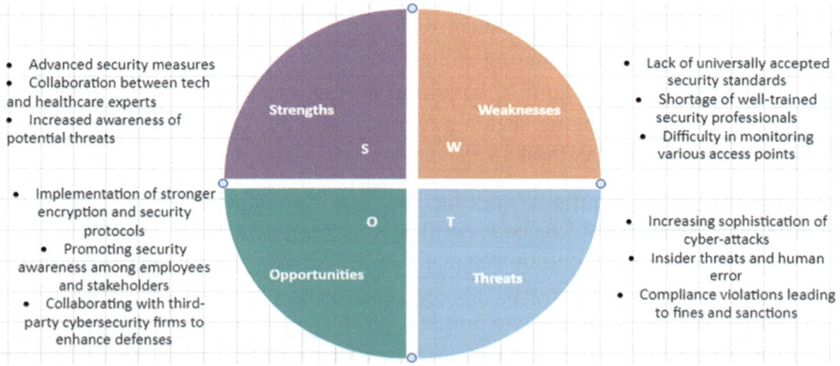

Fig. 7.2 Security threats in Meta-Health data

2. Insider Threats: Employees or contractors with access to Meta-Health data pose the biggest security threats purposely or even unknowingly. In fact, the importance of internal threats is hinged on either intention in committing acts of internal data theft or sabotage or in their failure to carelessly handle sensitive data, share passwords, or fail to follow the organizational rules regarding security.
3. Data Re-identification: Even with anonymization or de-identification efforts, there is a possibility that the subjects can still be identified through more sophisticated techniques used in data analysis and access to other data sources. This might risk the disclosure of personal health information that was considered well protected.
4. Third-Party Risks: There is a huge amount of data sharing in Meta-Health between third-party vendors, research partners, or sometimes healthcare providers. These can make the system vulnerable if their security practices are not up to mark, as there is a possibility of data leakage or unauthorized access.
5. Poor encryption of data or weakness in transmission protocols of health data can lead to the interception and tampering with health data during transmission or storage. Ensuring a high level of encryption standards and secure data transfer is very key to this risk mitigation.
6. Data Loss and Corruption: Technical failure, system crashes, and unintended deletion of data may lead to data loss or corruption. Hence, backup and recovery procedures should be implemented to avoid these risks and ensure integrity.
7. Compliance Violations: Poor compliance with data protection laws, such as GDPR or HIPAA, brings about a set of legal consequences and sensitive information being put at risk. In order to avoid compliance-related threats, regular audits and security practices must be carried out to maintain compliance with such regulations.
8. Phishing and Social Engineering: These are two of the main techniques that cybercriminals use to fool someone into giving away login credentials, which would directly compromise access to Meta-Health.
9. IoT device vulnerabilities: The increased use of IoT devices in the domain of health can introduce a security vulnerability if the devices are not properly secured. Exploits targeting IoT devices could offer unauthorized access to the data collected by the connected wearables or other devices.
10. Emerging Concerns: As technology is getting better with each passing day, new security threats and vulnerabilities emerge, which requires Meta-Health to further adapt continuously to be more watchful in protecting such data. It is of paramount importance that the newest threat intelligence and cybersecurity trends are watched for in maintaining updated data security (Bertino 2016).

The state-of-the-art technologies, strict access control, periodic security assessments, and regular employee training in Meta-Health protect the data and ensure its utilization securely in healthcare and research.

7.5.2 Common Attack Vectors: Ransomware, Phishing, and Insider Threats

The common attack vectors on the Meta-Health data are different ways as shown in Fig. 7.3 that cybercriminals attack in order to compromise the security of data. These include the following:

1. Ransomware: These are those attacks that involve encrypting a victim's information and later demand a ransom for the decryption key. Ransomware may lock major health information systems, leading to disrupted access to patient records, research data, and operational systems—major impacts on its operations and finances.
2. Phishing: These are types of attacks created to deceive a person into giving out personal data, such as login or personally identifiable information, through emails, messages, or websites. For Meta-Health, successful phishing means that unauthorized users are able to access health data systems, which could lead to more serious data breaches or identity theft.
3. Insider Threats: Insider threats are those that arise when employees, contractors, or other trusted individuals misuse their access to sensitive data. This is intentional, such as data theft or sabotage, or even unintentional, as in the mishandling of data or falling victim to social engineering attacks. This will expose patient confidentiality and integrity of data.
4. Malware: A set of malware is meant to get into a computer system to destruct or compromise systems, or even to thieve data. In Meta-Health, such malware can disrupt operations, corrupt data, or exfiltrate sensitive health information. Some examples of this class are viruses, worms, and Trojans.
5. Man-in-the-Middle Attacks: These refer to an attack in which communications between parties are intercepted and possibly altered in contents without the knowledge of the involved parties. For Meta-Health, such risks may violate both confidentiality and integrity for information in transit between health information systems or between patients and providers.

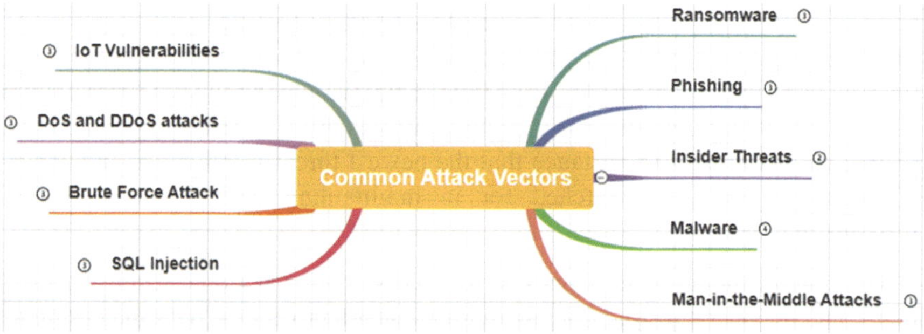

Fig. 7.3 Common attack vectors

6. SQL Injection: Manipulation or unauthorized access to data held within a database through the injection of malicious query codes. This may also lead to unauthorized access of patient records among other sensitive data stored in the Meta-Health.
7. It is an attack which involves the embedding of malicious scripts within a web application. These scripts execute when users access a particular web application. XSS in Meta-Health would facilitate the theft of credentials and session tokens of users by hackers, hence compromising the health data.
8. Brute Force Attack: Brute force is a disciplined process of trying several combinations of passwords or encryption keys until the right one is discovered. Such an attack within Meta-Health can be intrusive in its security mechanism if it does not have advanced ways of authenticating user accounts.
9. DoS and DDoS attacks are based on overloading systems or networks with so much network traffic that the services become unavailable. For the case of Meta-Health, for example, this may mean not being able to access or provide critical health information systems critical to patient care and operational activity.
10. IoT vulnerabilities: Since health organizations rely increasingly on the use of Internet of Things devices, any vulnerability within these devices can be used to gain unauthorized access to data or systems. This could include an attacker exploiting weaknesses in device security to compromise data collected by wearables or other connected health devices. The common attack vectors described demand a multilayered security approach: one that contains robust access controls, enhanced threat detection systems, periodic security training of employees, and sound incident response plans to minimize these varied risks and consequences of such attacks on Meta-Health data (Abomhara and Køien 2014).

7.5.3 Security Frameworks and Guidelines (e.g., NIST, ISO/IEC 27001)

Security frameworks and guidelines provide structured approaches to securing Meta-Health data. The recommended practices, standards, and protocols for the management of information security include notable frameworks and guidelines comprise the following:

- The NIST CSF was developed by the National Institute of Standards and Technology and provides a very holistic approach to cybersecurity risk management. It is organized around five core functions: Identify, Protect, Detect, Respond, and Recover. In this context, it will help Meta-Health in building and maintaining appropriate security posture by providing guidelines on the management of risk, protection of data, responding in cases of incidents, and recovery processes.

- ISO/IEC 27001 is an international standard that provides a formalized approach to the management of information security using an ISMS. The standard outlines the requirements for setting up, implementing, maintaining, and continually improving security controls to protect sensitive information. It includes a risk management process, which is important for Meta-Health in minimizing security risks that could compromise the confidentiality, integrity, and availability of health information.
  - ISO/IEC 27002: Building on ISO/IEC 27001, ISO/IEC 27002 provides guidance and best practices with regard to the implementation of controls. It includes topics on access control, encryption of data, and management of security incidents. In the case of Meta-Health, adherence to ISO/IEC 27002 would provide for a sound security policy and corresponding procedures, which would then safeguard patient data and guarantee compliance with the security standards.
  - General Data Protection Regulation: Although not one of the more traditional security frameworks, GDPR fills some critical guidelines necessary to help protect personal data within the European Union. Among these, some principles are data minimization, purpose limitation, and security measures that shall include appropriate technical and organizational controls for the protection of health data. In general, GDPR is the most important compliance and one that any organization operating or having entities in the EU should follow.
  - The Health Insurance Portability and Accountability Act (HIPAA) establishes regulations in the USA aimed at safeguarding patient health information. Specifically, the HIPAA Security Rule focuses on the protection of electronic health data through a framework of administrative, physical, and technical safeguards. Adhering to HIPAA mandates is essential for Meta-Health organizations to uphold the privacy and security of health-related information.
  - COBIT is an acronym for Control Objectives for Information and Related Technologies, a framework that is used to develop, implement, monitor, and improve IT governance and management practices. It provides a framework that guides the management of IT-related risks and assurance on information systems' integrity, something quite important to Meta-Health in ensuring security and efficient management of health information systems.

Although the main focus of the Payment Card Industry Data Security Standard PCI DSS is the protection of payment card information, it also provides numerous important security principles relevant to sensitive data protection in general. The requirements on data security, establishment of a vulnerability management framework, and implementation of strong access control policy are relevant to Meta-Health data protection.

7.6 Health Data Protection in Meta-Health

Data security at Meta-Health means amalgamating sources of varied data and high-end technology. In this regard, due attention should be drawn to sensitive health data protection. Strong encryption of data—both in transmission and in rest—strict access using role-based authentication and multifactor controls, data obfuscation techniques when analyzing sensitive information are just a few integral parts of good data security. It finds out the compliance vulnerabilities through continuous monitoring and periodic security audits. The lifecycle of the data will be taken cared of, from storing it appropriately to practicing proper deletions of it. Besides maintaining regulations such as HIPAA and GDPR, the company provides detailed training to employees, a clearly identified incident response plan, and a great role in the integrity of data, to avoid breaches with unauthorized access. These measures will abstract the Meta-Health data and will secure the data, not extracted effectively into the treatment and research work of the patients, and maintain the privacy and compliance standards.

7.6.1 Security Threats in Meta-Health Data

The range of security threats in Meta-Health data varies from such attacks, which bring a precarious effect on sensitive health information in terms of confidentiality, integrity, and availability. These include the following:

- Cyberattacks, more particularly ransomware, phishing, or malware that could be launched against the Meta-Health systems in search of illegal access, could also go as far as encrypting health data. The possible data breach incidents that might come out of such attacks can be too enormous in terms of loss in terms of patient information, financial cost, and possible erosion of trust.
- Insider Threats: The employees or contractors who have access to Meta-Health data are the biggest security threat in a deliberate or even inadvertent manner. Indeed, internal threats gain significance based on their intention to commit internal data theft or sabotage acts or in their failure to carelessly handle sensitive data, password sharing, or failing to follow organizational rules regarding security.
- Data Re-identification: Even when data is significantly anonymized or de-identified, it is still traceable through sophisticated analytical techniques or by accessing complementary sources of data. This could also pose a risk in unauthorized disclosure related to personal health information, which might be thought of as being very well protected.
- Third-Party Risks: Enormous data are shared within third-party vendors, research partners, or sometimes even healthcare providers in Meta-Health. If their security practices were below par, it would expose the system to great risks through data leakage or unauthorized access.

- Poor encryption of data or weak transmission protocols of health data may lead to intercepting and tampering with health data while in transit or during storage. To mitigate the risk, high standards of encryption should be ensured with secure transfer of data.
- Data Loss and Corruption: The failure of technology, system crashes, and accidental deletions can result in data loss or corruption. In light of these, backup and recovery processes will be implemented, which will prevent such risks and ensure integrity.
- Compliance Violations: Poor compliance with laws related to data protection—like GDPR, HIPAA—invites legal consequences, and sensitive information is brought at risk. In order to avoid threats that arise from compliance, one needs to conduct regular audits and follow security practices that keep them continuously compliant with such regulations.
- Phishing and social engineering would be major methods to be used by cyber adversaries to trick an individual out of his or her login credentials, with a direct finding of harming the access to Meta-Health.
- IoT Device Vulnerabilities: With the increased use of IoT devices in the health domain, it becomes a security vulnerability if the setup of devices is not secure. The exploits targeting IoT devices could promise to breach the data collected by the wearables or any other device that is connected, offering unauthorized access to it.

Emerging issues include the fact that, with exponential development in technology, each day poses new challenges to this security aspect, forcing Meta-Health to continuously evolve by being even more vigilant in the protection of such data. It will be all the more important that the most current threat intelligence and cybersecurity trends are being watched for in maintaining the most updated data security. It is in Meta-Health that state-of-the-art technologies, strict access control, periodic security assessments, and regular employee training protect the data for secure usage in healthcare and research purposes.

7.6.2 Common Attack Vectors: Ransomware, Phishing, and Insider Threats

By common attack vectors, it generally means those different points from which cybercriminals start an attack with the intention of compromising the security of data. Some of the common attack vectors on the data in Meta-Health are as follows:

1. Ransomware: The attacks that involve encrypting a victim's information involve leaving out more innuendo and demanding a ransom in exchange for the decryption key. Ransomware can lock major health information systems,

hence hindering access to patient files, research data, and operational systems—major impacts on its operations and finances.

2. Phishing: Types of attacks created to deceive a person into giving away personal information, be it login or personally identifiable information, sent through emails, messages, or websites. In Meta-Health, successful phishing would mean that unauthorized persons have infiltrated the health systems, with potential consequences of more serious data breaches and identity theft.
3. Insider Threats: Insider threats are considered the actions made by employees, contractors, or any other trusted party who misuse their access to sensitive data. It may be intentional, including examples such as data theft or sabotage, or even unintentional, such as mishandling of data or unintentional social engineering attacks. This will result in the breach of patient confidentiality and integrity of information.
4. Malware: A collection of malware is designed to penetrate a computer system to destroy or incapacitate the system and, at times, to cause theft. Through Meta-Health, the consequences can be from disrupted services to damaged data and leaking sensitive health information. The class includes—but is not limited to—viruses, worms, and Trojans.
5. Man-in-the-Middle Attack: These describe an attack where the communication between the two parties is eavesdropped and possibly altered in contents without the knowledge of the parties involved. It is presumed that the possible Meta-Health risks may violate confidentiality and integrity of information in transit among health information systems or between patients/providers.
6. SQL Injection: This is a form of knocking a database by the insertion of malicious query codes that may affect the data stored in the database. This could also lead to unauthorized access to patient records and other sensitive data stored in Meta-Health.

It is an attack that extracts a script from a web application. A functional application executes these scripts when a user launches a specific web application. Having XSS in Meta-Health would allow the hackers to steal the users' credentials and the users' session tokens, thereby allowing them access to health data.

Brute Force Attack: Brute force is a disciplined process of trying several combinations of passwords or encryption keys until the right one is discovered. In such an attack within Meta-Health, it can be intrusive in its security mechanism if it does not have advanced ways of authenticating user accounts.

DoS and DDoS are basically overloading systems or networks with so much network traffic that services become unavailable. For example, in the case of Meta-Health, this would mean not being able to access or provide critical health information systems fundamental to patient care and operational activity.

7.7 Meta-Health: Risk Management

Risk management in Meta-Health is such an important process. It requires the identification, assessment, and mitigation of risks associated with sensitive health data handling. It begins with the determination of various types of threats that may emanate from cyberattacks, insider threats, or technical failures. Those risks are then assessed for their likelihood and potential impact, thus helping organizations prioritize their efforts in responding. The mitigation strategies involve the use of encrypting technologies, effective access controls, and regular security training to reduce or eradicate the risks. Continuous monitoring comes in handy to ensure strategies for the management of risk keep up to date and change with emerging threats. Incident response plans are designed to contain and control security incidents. Regulatory requirements, such as those by HIPAA and GDPR, are followed in efforts to minimize legal and regulatory risks. Effective risk communication ensures that all parties involved understand their role in data protection, while the risk transfer mechanisms, including cybersecurity insurance, can provide fiscal protection. This requires a continuous reevaluation and update of the risk management framework to meet evolving challenges and consider enhancements to improve data security overall, protection of Meta-Health data, and confidence for the patients and stakeholders involved (Zhang et al. 2023).

7.7.1 Risk Assessment and Threat Modeling

It is considered that risk assessment and threat modeling are base-level components of the broad Meta-Health risk management strategy, a process that identifies, develops, and fixes all possible securities that could potentially compromise sensitive health information. Risk assessment is the process of methodically identifying and evaluating the potential risks that may affect systems and data. Identification of assets included information about patients, health records, and IT infrastructure, while identification of vulnerabilities and threats means cyberattacks, failures of systems, or human mistakes. All identified risks should be assessed for their likelihood and potential impact by means of tools such as risk matrices and quantitative analyses. Its scope is to rank risks according to their seriousness, in order for the organization to take appropriate action and address first the most vital threats. Regularly, risk assessments enable an organization to keep pace with changes in technology, regulations, and threat landscapes.

Threat modeling basically complements risk assessment through the understanding and analysis of the probable threats and attack vectors peculiar to Meta-Health. It involves the making of models and diagrams that show system architecture, data flow, and interaction with various components. The benefit of threat modeling identifies system weaknesses an attacker might use to gain access, for example, in data transmission vulnerabilities or poor implementation of access controls.

The approaches like Spoofing, Tampering, Repudiation, Information Disclosure, Denial of Service, and Elevation of Privilege (STRIDE) and Process for Attack Simulation and Threat Analysis (PASTA) enabled systematic detection and documentation of the potential threats. These simulations will thus allow different organizations to come up with specific security interventions and incident response plans in an effort or intent to mitigate the identified threats by artificially running through attacks under various scenarios and their impacts on health data. Taken together, risk assessment and threat modeling present a big-picture look at the security landscape for Meta-Health, in which organizations can prepare for risks, deliver appropriate security controls, and protect sensitive health information from ever-changing threats.

7.7.2 *Vulnerability Management and Incident Response*

It would involve vulnerability management and incident response in securing data for Meta-Health against security breaches for quick recovery upon incidents. These two related processes entail determining weaknesses within systems and taking remedial action while responding effectively to security events. The security vulnerabilities will be identified in Meta-Health systems through a structured process for vulnerability management. This consists of regular scanning and vulnerability testing to be able to identify the weak points in software, hardware, and network configurations. Some of the tools used in vulnerability scanning and penetration test methodologies involve the use of antique software, other misconfigurations, and unpatched systems. Once identified, the next step is to assess vulnerabilities in terms of severity and impact. It allows organizations to prioritize remediation efforts through patching, updating, or reconfiguring the systems with the most critical vulnerabilities first. Continuous monitoring along with periodic assessments assists in early actions against newly emerging threats and supports their environment in a secured way.

Incident Response: This is the methodical process or procedure used to manage and mitigate the effects of security incidents when they occur. An effective incident response plan outlines procedures for detecting, containing, and eradicating security breaches. This involves defining the roles and responsibilities of members belonging to the incident response team, developing communication and contact plans, and creating procedures for collecting, analyzing, and recovering data. Key components of incident response include the following:

- Detection and Analysis: Prompt detection and analysis to establish the nature, scope, and impact of the security incidents. This includes monitoring systems for unusual activities, log analysis, and the use of forensic tools to comprehend in detail the attack.

- Containment: Immediate action initiated to limit the spread of the incident and prevent further damage. This may involve isolation of affected systems, disabling compromised accounts, or blocking malicious network traffic.
- Eradication procedure is the removal of the reasons of the incident—for example, malware deletion, closure of vulnerability, or fixing the problem that allowed some breach.
- Recovery means restoring compromised systems and services to normal working condition and ensuring the correction of all detected weaknesses. It includes checking the integrity of the systems, data restoration from backup, and verification of effective operation of security measures. Review following the incident: Do a critical analysis of the incident to understand, specifically, what happened, how it was handled, and how it can be improved upon. Document the lessons learned and revise the security policies, procedures, and incident response plan accordingly. Through the integration of vulnerability management and incident response, Meta-Health organizations are able to proactively identify and mitigate potential security vulnerabilities while remaining equipped to respond adeptly to incidents. This approach would ensure the systematic elimination of the identified security risks to maintain secure data and minimize disruptions and improve in general resilience and security of health information systems.

7.7.3 *Mitigation Strategies*

It is only by taking those vulnerabilities and threats that could probably be exploited—their vulnerability and the possible risk or threat level represented by the vulnerability—into account that, with mitigation strategies, the security of Meta-Health data can be assured. This strategy includes various controls and measures that decrease the possible impact of the security risks, thereby enhancing general health information system security. Noted as being the most critical among these are as follows:

Access Control: It helps in the prevention of unauthorized access to sensitive health data by any unauthorized individual; in other words, it is also granted to only those to whom data are intended. In this regard, role-based access control or adhering to the principle of least privilege and multifactor authentication access may be in order.

Data Encryption: The data encryption will secure the data at rest and in transit against unauthorized access and breach. This will be done using the most recent encryption algorithms such as AES, using the latest secure communication protocols, for example, TLS, to ensure the security of the data in transmission.

1. Patch management should be a regular procedure; updating the software, applications, and systems with security patches keeps the door closed to known vulnerabilities. Develop a robust patch management process updating

those dealing with critical fixes for quick application, reducing the risks attributed by security defects.

2. Network Security: Network access control through the security deployed in the network, such as firewalls, intrusion detection systems, and intrusion prevention systems, works against unauthorized access and cyberattacks. Such configuration of security is related to network segmentation, which helps reduce attack surfaces.
3. Security Awareness Training: Routine training is important for staff to develop identification skills and an understanding of how to act in case of a perceived threat, be it a phishing attack or social engineering. Educated staff are prone to a lesser risk of attack, with better compliance in adhering to security best practices.
4. Vulnerability management involves the routine assessment of vulnerabilities and penetration testing to ensure that security weaknesses are identified. Rapid discovery and remediation of problems, following monitoring against emerging threats, builds the area into a proactive approach to vulnerability management.
5. Incident Response Planning: The development and maintenance of the incident response plan implies that in case there is a security incident with an organization, then the responses and recoveries can be effectively dealt with. It should cover procedures for incident detection and containment and outline databases for the eradication/mitigation and should outline clear roles and responsibilities within the response team.
6. Backup and recovery of data: Data are the most critical health-restoring information. Therefore, it is the development and implementation of scheduled data backup and restoration processes that guarantee ways of restoring health-critical information in the event of its loss, destruction, or corruption—namely, even in a ransomware attack. Periodic testing of backup solutions will be carried out to ensure the integrity of data and availability.
7. Regulatory Compliance: This is where meeting regulatory requirements, including HIPAA and GDPR, as derived from all related data protection legislation, is ensured so that security practices are all legal for protecting patient data. Regular audits and updated assessments will keep them on track with compliance and block possible gaps.
8. Physical Security: Securing data centers and IT infrastructure physically from unauthorized access along with other environmental perils. Major components of physical security involve access controls, the use of surveillance systems at the premises, and appropriate facility management practices.
9. Third-Party Risk Management: Third-party vendors and partners represent security risks that need to be quantified and minimized. The corresponding activities involve the action of executing security assessments, assurances on third parties, establishment of contracts through which security responsibilities are clearly defined, and others.

Thus, the organizations participating in Meta-Health would be able to reduce the likelihood of occurrence and actual consequence of security incidents on sensitive health data through the adoption of a security risk mitigation strategy whereby they could ensure a secure and resilient health information environment.

7.8 Case Studies of Security Breaches in Meta-Health

The different cases involving data breaches in Meta-Health present various issues and also outcomes on the weaknesses of data defense systems; however, they also shed light on valuable lessons that can be further taken into consideration for fortifying security methodologies. The above discussion throws huge light on how such breaches are really possible, the outcomes that result from it towards organizations and patients, and the ways similar incidents can be avoided in the future.

7.8.1 Case Study: 2020 Ransomware Attack on Scripps Health

In May 2020, Scripps Health, one of the biggest healthcare systems in San Diego, was pummelled by a huge ransomware attack. The attackers encrypted the organization's data, in turn breaking the functionality of the hospitals, including patient care services and access to EHRs.

Effect: The attack resulted in a long-standing disruption in hospital services, including appointment and surgery cancellations. On the other hand, it encrypted details of the patients in such a way that it was untraceable; hence, some operations were compromised that possibly set back the attention extended to the patients.

Scripps Health partnered with cybersecurity experts to cover and thereby minimize the impacts of the breach. The facility took emergency measures in attempting to restore service to its patients and kept open communications about the same with the patients. Restoration was done at a system-by-system manner to be sure of integrity; this event also led to a deep analysis and enhancement of cyber strategies (Singh and Malhotra 2023).

Learning from Incident: The data breach was evidence that consistent data backup was necessary, a well-prepared comprehensive incident response strategy, and the most important of all, training programs for the employees to identify and mitigate phishing effectively.

7.8.2 *Case Study: 2015 Anthem Inc. Data Breach*

In February 2015, Anthem Inc., one of the largest health insurance companies in America, reported that its data had been exposed, including personal identifying information about nearly 78.8 million individuals. Structures involved in causing such incidents have been specified as advanced cyberattack that jeopardized firm data.

Impact: The data stolen included such information as names, birthdates, and Social Security numbers. People were most worried about identity theft and fraud.

Anthem implemented extra security that involved much more robust encryption algorithms and higher monitoring ability. Further, the company offered credit monitoring programs to those who were affected and worked with the investigations of regulators.

Lessons Learnt: It pinpointed the strong data encryption, proactivity in identifying threats, and monitoring systems. It also emphasized timely communication and support to the affected individuals.

7.8.3 *Case Analysis: The 2017 WannaCry Ransomware Incident*

Incident: The ransomware attack was unleashed in May 2017, and it managed to infect a lot of its targets worldwide. Among its impact was the interference with the normal operations of several healthcare providers under the UK National Health Service—affecting this sector in a huge way. This debut ransomware encrypted the files and demanded payments—in Bitcoin, of course.

Impact: Main consequences of the cyberattack—it obscured NHS operations through appointment and surgical procedure cancelations. It deeply disrupted several hospitals and healthcare centers, leading to the postponement of patient treatments and the disruption of their operation.

The NHS handled that with turning off involved devices that are attacked by the ransomware behavior to contain the spread and restoring from back up to bring services back to operational status before implementing a security update in at-risk devices to prevent the next wave of attacks.

Lessons Learnt: The Ransomware attack pinpointed the exact desperate need to upgrade software at the earliest possible time and effectively managed available security patches. As much as it showed the need and importance of conducting regular data backups, it also pointed out the same for comprehensive incident response strategies.

7.8.4 *Case Study: 2021 Data Breach at University of Virginia Health System*

Event: In June 2021, the University of Virginia Health System experienced an event relating to the breach of patient records, facilitated by the unauthorized actions of an employee. As a result, there was a breach of patients' information that was confidential, being personal health and medical information.

Consequence: It has affected a very large number of patients, which raised concerns about the privacy and use of medical records. Unauthorized access was detected by internal review. The health system informed impacted patients and implemented further security settings to prevent similar cases in the future. The health system conducted an extensive investigation into the matter and reviewed its access and monitoring practices.

Lessons Learnt: There should be strong access controls, with systematic audit and continuous monitoring of the activities of employees, to prevent and detect unauthorized access to this information classified as confidential. The case studies give key messages on how sensitive the security measures to be carried out are, these being processes like encryption, access controls, updating, and responding to incident planning. These also provide a clue on the necessity of continuous improvement and vigilance in preserving Meta-Health data against threats.

7.9 Future Directions and Challenges

Emerging trends and challenges in Meta-Health continue to take shape on the landscape of data privacy and security at a time of continued technological change and evolving methodologies in healthcare. The second most important trend is deeper integration of AI and machine learning in health. While this promises new benefits related to diagnosis and personalized therapies, it equally presents new security risks in manipulation or hacking of the AI models themselves. Interoperable health devices and proliferation of IoMT therefore bring with them volumes of information generated, contributing to an increased attack surface. It sets a developing trend that calls for an increase in more sophisticated measures against the vulnerability of those devices. Moreover, telemedicine and RPM create concerns regarding the protection of data transmitted over perhaps insecure networks and compliance with diverse privacy requirements within many jurisdictions. While the regulations are becoming evolved—say, GDPR and HIPAA—companies have to sail through the evolving set of compliances, integrating new technologies while keeping the bar high for data protection standards. The sophistication of cyberattacks—from ransomware to focused phishing campaigns—demands a constant adaptation of security strategies in investment in sophisticated threat detection and response capabilities. Needless to say, this interoperability of systems and sharing of data for both research and care has to be balanced against strenuous protection of privacy so as not to allow unauthorized access and misuse of confidential data. These future trends and challenges put a demand for a proactive and adaptive cybersecurity approach through continuous risk assessments, investments in advanced security technologies, and a high level of commitment to patient data protection in the continuously changing digital environment (Said et al. 2024).

7.9.1 Future Directions in Privacy and Security Technologies

The future of privacy and security technologies for Meta-Health will thus be quite different, enabled by technological advancements and shifting regulatory environments. Quantum encryption, for example, will provide unprecedented levels of security by harnessing the power of quantum mechanics at its core to protect information from potential future quantum computing threats. Blockchain technology is increasingly recognized for its capability in guaranteeing data integrity and transparency through setting up unalterable transaction records that could enhance health data exchanges in security and traceability. Embedding PET will, among others, cover secure multiparty computation and homomorphic encryption to enable processing and analysis without disclosure of individual data points, which will keep the privacy while exploiting the valuable insights. AI and ML will be crucial in the detection and response to threats, given their capability of identifying patterns and anomalies in large datasets; again, this will also require effective safeguards against adversarial attacks on AI systems themselves. Zero-trust architectures will really flip the paradigm of security frameworks because, by default, no user or device can be trusted; thus, there is a need for constant verification and authorization to sensitive information. As regulatory demands on secure data handling continue to evolve, privacy-by-design principles will be instrumental in embedding these throughout the creation and deployment of emerging technologies. Further, it is envisioned that advances in biometric security will continue to afford increasingly sophisticated modes of authentication that include behavioral biometric and multimodal authentications toward twin goals of hardened access controls and reduced risk of unauthorized access. These possible future developments certainly put the proactive approach to the fore in matters of privacy and security in Meta-Health through innovating and laying strict protections to guard sensitive health information moving on continuous digital shift.

7.9.2 Challenges in Adopting Privacy and Security Best Practices

Various other challenges and problems beset the best practices for privacy and security, showing the overall challenge involved in protecting sensitive health data across a constantly changing environment. Perhaps the biggest challenge is that there is increasingly more speed required when it comes to ever-evolving threats and methods of cyberattacks, and sometimes that means needing updates in security protocols more and more constantly, constant staff training, and so on and so forth. For example, the adoption of new technologies, such as IoT devices and AI systems, further exacerbates the challenge in security management, as technologies come with a long list of vulnerabilities and require very specialized security measures. These are even complemented by challenges in compliance with diversified and dynamic regulations because organizations have to consider a number of national and international laws on data protection, varied in both requirements and standards, leading to inconsistencies and administrative burdens. This is a very challenging goal, balancing this tension between the need for interoperability and sharing of data by different healthcare systems, without consideration of data privacy, contributing to seamless and effective care for the patients. Resource constraints in small budgets and personnel are potential barriers toward being able to do security well, especially for smaller healthcare providers. Thirdly, user education and awareness become critical because, at the end of it all, human error is one of the big vulnerabilities, and high levels of training and awareness are fraught and resource-intensive tasks. Lastly, there is also the problem of dealing with the vulnerabilities of legacy systems since most of the health organizations run on older systems that are pretty difficult to secure and integrate with modern security technologies. It requires an integrated approach to investing in sophisticated technologies, a strong strategy that guarantees compliance, and ongoing enhancements in privacy and security practices that reassure trust.

7.10 Conclusion

The conclusion is that in the Meta-Health data-privacy-and-security landscape, unparalleled advancement coexists with a challenge. Huge dependence on digital technologies with widely connected devices places pressure on the need for protection of highly sensitive health information in healthcare systems. This offers promising avenues to improve data security and privacy through integration with leading-edge technologies such as AI, blockchain, and quantum encryption. On the other hand, these advances introduce new vulnerabilities and require continuous development and adaptation of security strategies. Performing the eternal balancing act between data interoperability and the strict protection of data, understanding and working within constantly changing regulatory environments, and the peculiar challenges provided by emerging technologies go hand in hand in perpetuation solid security regimes. For this reason, advanced threat detection should be built, comprehensive risk management monitored, and users educated if organizations are to protect patient data. In sum, health providers can help safeguard sensitive health information, foster patient trust in this regard, and promote the advancement of a secure and resilient Meta-Health environment by adopting an active and adaptive approach to privacy and security. It is in addressing such challenges and assuming future directions of technology that the fullest benefits of digital health innovations will be realized without compromising the security and privacy of patient data.

References

Abomhara M, Køien GM (2014) Security and privacy in the Internet of Things: current status and open issues. In: 2014 international conference on privacy and security in mobile systems (PRISMS), Aalborg, Denmark, pp 1–8. https://doi.org/10.1109/PRISMS.2014.6970594

Abouelmehdi K, Beni-Hessane A, Khaloufi H (2018) Big healthcare data: preserving security and privacy. J Big Data 5:1. https://doi.org/10.1186/s40537-017-0110-7

Bertino E (2016) Data security and privacy: concepts, approaches, and research directions. In: 2016 IEEE 40th annual computer software and applications conference (COMPSAC), Atlanta, GA, USA, pp 400–407. https://doi.org/10.1109/COMPSAC.2016.89

Said A, Yahyaoui A, Abdellatif T (2024) HIPAA and GDPR compliance in IoT healthcare systems. In: Mosbah M et al (eds) Advances in model and data engineering in the digitalization era. MEDI 2023. Communications in computer and information science, vol 2071. Springer, Cham. https://doi.org/10.1007/978-3-031-55729-3_16

Singh K, Malhotra D (2023) Meta-health: learning-to-learn (meta-learning) as a next generation of deep learning exploring healthcare challenges and solutions for rare disorders: a systematic analysis. Arch Computat Methods Eng 30:4081–4112. https://doi.org/10.1007/s11831-023-09927-8

Watters PA (2023) Cyber threats (and opportunities). In: Counterintelligence in a cyber world. Springer, Cham. https://doi.org/10.1007/978-3-031-35287-4_3

Zhang T, Shen J, Lai C-F, Ji S, Ren Y (2023) Multi-server assisted data sharing supporting secure deduplication for metaverse healthcare systems. Future Gen Comput Syst 140:299–310

Chapter 8
Mimicking Healthcare in Meta-Health

8.1 Introduction

8.1.1 Overview of Meta-Health

In the past few decades, the healthcare industry has seen enormous advancements and changes brought about by advances in technology. One such innovative concept is Meta-Health, which integrates the metaverse with healthcare to transform the availability and delivery of medical services. Meta-Health represents a significant advancement in healthcare by offering virtual and tactile experiences that imitate typical healthcare venues in a digital setting. Stated differently, Meta-Health can be characterized as follows:

8.1.1.1 What Is Meta-Health?

The integration of immersive technology such as virtual reality and augmented reality (AR) into healthcare operations is referred to as "Meta-Health" (Lee 2022). The healthcare sector delivers exciting and comprehensive medical interactions that enable customers, medical professionals, and other stakeholders to engage in virtual environments that mimic actual medical environments by harnessing the potential of the metaverse.

8.1.1.2 The Potential of Meta-Health

Meta-Health offers great possibilities to improve the experience of patients and transform the manner in which healthcare is provided. By providing simulated environments that closely resemble actual healthcare facilities, Meta-Health makes it possible to conduct training sessions, distant consultations, and better medical

S. Vyas et al., *Meta-Health*, https://doi.org/10.1007/978-981-96-5844-2_8

scenarios (Ullah et al. 2023). It can remove time, setting, and availability barriers in the healthcare sector, opening up new possibilities for individualized and efficient care.

8.1.1.3 Advantages of Meta-Health

Meta-Health offers several advantages that traditional healthcare institutions might not be able to match. Among these are as follows:

Enhanced Accessibility

People in rural locations or with limited mobility can utilize Meta-Health's services from the comfort of their homes, negating the need for physical travel. Meta-Health also removes geographical limitations to promote accessibility (Suh et al. 2023; Bansal et al. 2022).

Realistic Simulations

Healthcare workers can practice complex operations, polish their abilities, and earn vital experience in a secure and monitored virtual environment using Meta-Health's highly realistic medical simulators (Suh et al. 2023; Al-Ghaili et al. 2022).

Personalized and Engaging Experiences

Meta-Health virtual environments are customized to meet the needs of individual patients, providing individualized healthcare experiences (Mourtzis 2023). Patients can actively participate in their healthcare journey by using immersive technologies and interactive simulations. This can help patients learn more about self-care, which will enhance their comprehension and compliance (Chengoden et al. 2023).

Cost-Efficiency

By reducing the need for physical infrastructure, streamlining procedures, and maximizing resource use, Meta-Health offers the potential to lower healthcare expenditures. It might also lower the expense of travel for medical appointments (Sprenger and Schwaninger 2021).

8.1.1.4 Ethical Considerations

Meta-Health has many benefits, but it also brings up ethical issues that should be taken into mind (Thomason 2021; Waqas 2022; Singh and Malhotra 2023; De Abreu Lourenco et al. 2017). These include maintaining the integrity and quality of virtual healthcare services, protecting patient privacy and data security, obtaining informed consent for virtual procedures, and guaranteeing equitable access for all people, regardless of their socioeconomic status or level of technological proficiency (De Abreu Lourenco et al. 2017).

In summary, Meta-Health is a cutting-edge strategy for bringing modern healthcare up to date through the use of a virtual environment. It accomplishes this by utilizing the metaverse's capabilities to replicate traditional healthcare environments in a virtual environment. Removing obstacles related to location and accessibility has the potential to significantly improve patient health and alter healthcare services. Nonetheless, ethical issues must be addressed, and Meta-Health must be responsibly included in the healthcare system. We will examine many facets of Meta-Health and its influence on the healthcare sector as we proceed through this chapter.

8.1.2 Importance of Mimicking Healthcare

In the context of the transforming healthcare landscape, the idea of replicating healthcare in Meta-Health is quite important (Waqas 2022). Meta-Health wants to create a digital version of the traditional healthcare experience by utilizing virtual technologies. This has various advantages that emphasize how crucial it is to imitate healthcare:

8.1.2.1 Enhanced Patient Engagement

Patients at Meta-Health can actively contribute to their healthcare advancement through the use of mimicking healthcare (Suh et al. 2023). Patients can make more educated decisions about their health by using interactive experiences and simulations to better understand their diseases and treatment alternatives. Improved patient satisfaction and better health outcomes may result from greater involvement.

8.1.2.2 Training and Education Advancements

Professionals can improve their abilities, expertise, and proficiency with Meta-Health's educational programs on a virtual platform (Thomason 2021). Realistic practice scenarios made possible by simulated environments help medical professionals hone their skills, pick up new ones, and stay current, all of which contribute to providing higher-quality healthcare services overall.

8.1.2.3 Accessibility and Geographical Conditions

By imitating the healthcare system, we can get around geographic restrictions and improve access to healthcare services (Thomason 2021). Patients who live in remote areas will benefit from this since it will make it easier for them to get healthcare services. This lessens the need for people to move around as much, increases healthcare equity, and guarantees that everyone can access timely, appropriate care wherever they constitute (Gopika et al. 2022).

8.1.2.4 Cost-Effectiveness and Efficiency

Virtual healthcare platforms can lower costs for both patients and healthcare providers, and Meta-Health has the potential to do so by eliminating the need for physical infrastructure and optimizing processes. Furthermore, remote monitoring and virtual consultations can cut down on pointless hospital stays, saving money and improving healthcare effectiveness.

8.2 Objectives of the Chapter

The goal of Meta-Health's chapter on imitating healthcare is to give readers an in-depth knowledge of how the metaverse is being incorporated into healthcare and how new business models are emerging. This chapter's main goals are as follows:

8.2.1 Explore the Evolution of Meta-Health

This chapter will explore how the use of immersive and virtual technologies is changing healthcare services. Presenting opportunities for innovative patient care, medical education, and healthcare.

8.2.2 New Business Models in Meta-Health

The chapter will discuss cutting-edge business models and how they provide healthcare. It will examine every virtual platform for healthcare, telemedicine services, marketplaces for healthcare, medical education and training, data analytics and insights, and virtual experiences for health and wellness.

8.2.3 Key Considerations for Meta-Health Business Models

This chapter will highlight critical elements that should be taken into account when creating and executing business plans in the field of Meta-Health. We will concentrate on analyzing the market and determining the target market, evaluating the infrastructure and technology needs, and comprehending regulatory and legal compliance in Meta-Health business models.

8.2.4 Examine Challenges and Future Outlook

The chapter will list potential difficulties and roadblocks to the adoption of new business models in Meta-Health. We will also talk about prospective developments and future trends in Meta-Health business models, offering insights into how the virtual healthcare industry is changing.

8.3 Concepts and Principles of Mimicking Healthcare

8.3.1 Definition and Scope of Mimicking Healthcare

In the context of Meta-Health, mimicking healthcare entails reproducing and modeling a number of conventional healthcare components in a virtual and immersive environment (Bansal et al. 2022; Thomason 2021; Bashir et al. 2023). It includes recreating healthcare experiences, interactions, and services through the use of cutting-edge technologies like mixed reality (MR), augmented reality (AR), virtual reality (VR), and other digital platforms.

The scope of healthcare mimicking is wide and includes many aspects of the healthcare ecosystem comprised of the following points:

8.3.1.1 Virtual Consultations

Through virtual consultations with medical professionals, such as nurses, physiotherapists, doctors, and other support staff, patients can receive diagnoses, discuss treatment options, and voice concerns about their health without physically visiting their doctor. This technology is known as "mimicking healthcare." This entails reproducing, albeit in a digital setting, the dynamics, and face-to-face interactions of consultation that occur in real life (Mendell et al. 2019).

8.3.1.2 Remote Monitoring and Telemedicine

Patients' health data, health parameters, and medical conditions can be remotely monitored through the use of wearable devices, sensors, and connected technologies in healthcare simulation. Healthcare professionals are able to monitor patients' health and provide guidance in real-time. Geographical barriers are removed when healthcare services are delivered remotely through telemedicine solutions (Singh and Malhotra 2023; Jeddi and Bohr 2020).

8.3.1.3 Virtual Training and Medical Education

Training and education for healthcare professionals is another area where imitation of healthcare is practised (Kneebone 2003). Medical students, residents, and even seasoned professionals can practice surgeries, procedures, and critical care scenarios in a safe and controlled environment by using virtual environments (Graafland et al. 2012). It also provides chances for skill improvement, lifelong learning, and staying aware of the most recent developments in medicine.

8.3.1.4 Digital Health Records and Data Analytics

The idea of "imitating healthcare" encompasses data analysis, health record management, and digitization (Berros et al. 2023). Electronic health records (EHRs) make patient health records accessible and safe for data storage, which promotes easy coordination and communication between healthcare providers (Berros et al. 2023; Griffith et al. 2019; Hemingway et al. 2018). Furthermore, the identification of diagnostic patterns, the support of clinical decision-making, the extraction of insights from massive datasets, and the improvement of patient care are all made possible by data analytics.

8.3.1.5 Virtual Health and Wellness Experiences

Experiences in virtual reality can be created to encourage mindfulness, stress reduction, relaxation, and therapeutic interventions (Bansal et al. 2022; Benedicta et al. 2020; Amini et al. 2013). These immersive programs provide a fresh method for addressing holistic care, mental health, and well-being (Amini et al. 2013). By encompassing the users' experiences with health and wellness, these services contribute to a larger cause.

The field of healthcare mimicking is constantly expanding due to technological advancements and the discovery of new information. By utilizing the sophisticated capabilities of the metaverse, this seeks to duplicate the fundamental components of conventional healthcare.

8.3.2 *Key Concepts and Principles*

8.3.2.1 Virtualization of Healthcare Services

Virtual healthcare services involve in designing and creating digital representations and simulations of various healthcare processes and activities (Kasurinen 2017). By utilizing technologies such as virtual reality (VR), augmented reality (AR), and telemedicine platforms, services can be delivered remotely and accessed virtually.

8.3.2.2 Replication of Physical Health Systems

Mimicking healthcare aims to replicate and redesign healthcare systems in a virtual environment. This development requires understanding the infrastructure, workflows, and dynamics of traditional healthcare settings, such as hospitals, clinics, and medical facilities (Singer et al. 2015). By closely mimicking, we can maintain familiarity and continuity in the delivery of care.

8.3.2.3 User Experience and Engagement

A key principle in mimicking healthcare is the emphasis on user experience and engagement (Kuo et al. 2011). To accomplish this objective, user interfaces virtual environments and interactive tools are designed to enhance engagement, facilitate ease of use, and provide a sense of presence within the virtual healthcare setting (Johansen 2019). This principle ensures that the digital experience closely aligns with the expectations and needs of users, fostering a positive and effective healthcare encounter.

8.3.2.4 Personalization and Customization

The digital nature of the metaverse allows for tailoring healthcare experiences and services to individual needs and preferences (Richardson 2012; Dingler et al. 2021). Through data analytics, patient profiles, and personalized algorithms, healthcare interactions can be tailored according to the user needs and treatment plans (Chen et al. 2023). This concept promotes patient-centered care and improves outcomes by addressing individualized healthcare needs within the virtual environment.

8.3.2.5 Integration of Real-Time Communication and Collaboration

In mimicking healthcare, real-time communication and collaboration tools are integrated into the virtual environment to enable seamless interaction and exchange of information among healthcare professionals (He et al. 2021). Here healthcare providers can consult, share patient data, discuss cases, and collaborate on treatment plans in real time, regardless of geographical location. This principle enhances interdisciplinary collaboration and enables efficient healthcare decision-making (Che et al. 2015; Veldwijk et al. 2017).

8.3.2.6 Security and Privacy

Security and privacy of the patient data in the digital environment is highly important. At this level, we emphasize on robust security measures, encryption protocols, and adherence to privacy regulations to ensure the confidentiality and integrity of patient data (Vadlamudi 2022; Malhotra et al. 2021). This principle ensures that data within the virtual environment maintain the highest standards of privacy and security, without sacrificing the patient's information to anyone (Lenger 2022; Aziz 2018; Zainab et al. 2022).

8.3.2.7 Integration of Machine Learning and Artificial Intelligence

Another key concept in mimicking healthcare is the integration of machine learning (ML) and artificial intelligence (AI) technologies (Chavda et al. 2023). Both ML and AI play a crucial role in analyzing vast amounts of healthcare data, identifying patterns, and making predictions to support clinical decision-making and improve patient outcomes. The information provided by Ngiam and Khor (2019) the ML and AI algorithms can help in better predictions and assist in diagnosing diseases, suggesting treatment plans, and monitoring patient progress (Chavda et al. 2023; Ngiam and Khor 2019; Ellahham et al. 2020). By integrating ML and AI into the virtual healthcare environment, healthcare providers can leverage intelligent systems to enhance accuracy, efficiency, and effectiveness in healthcare delivery.

8.3.2.8 Simulation and Modeling Techniques

Simulation and modeling techniques are essential in mimicking healthcare within the Meta-Health framework (Nawawi et al. 2021; Roufaeel n.d.). These techniques are the backbone of the Meta-Health universe, involved in creating virtual representations and simulations of healthcare scenarios, procedures, and systems. Simulation and modeling techniques also enable the testing and optimization of healthcare processes and workflows, leading to improved efficiency and patient safety (Mans et al. 2013; Alwasel et al. 2021). Also, through realistic simulations, healthcare providers can practice and refine their skills at their convenience, as the information is always available online, this also helps to evaluate different treatment strategies and assess the impact of interventions in a controlled and risk-free environment.

In mimicking healthcare, ML and AI technologies as well as simulation and modeling techniques work in synergy to create highly intelligent virtual environments where realistic healthcare scenarios can be simulated, analyzed, and optimized. The integration of ML and AI enhances the capabilities of simulations by introducing intelligent agents, dynamic responses, and personalized interactions based on patient data and clinical guidelines.

8.4 Applications of Mimicking Healthcare in Meta-Health

8.4.1 Virtual Patient Care

Virtual patient care is a significant application of mimicking healthcare within the Meta-Health framework. The following are key applications within virtual patient care:

8.4.1.1 Telemedicine and Remote Consultations

Mimicking healthcare enables the utilization of telemedicine services and remote consultations. By utilizing video conferencing, chat platforms, and other communication technologies, we offer a high level of telehealth facilities (Senbekov et al. 2020). Virtual platforms will provide a secure and convenient means for patients to seek medical services without the need for physical visits. This approach is quite helpful for those who live in remote areas.

8.4.1.2 Virtual Clinics and Hospitals

Virtual clinics and hospitals can be created in Meta-Health to replicate the functions of physical healthcare facilities (Bansal et al. 2022; Mourtzis 2023; Chengoden et al. 2023). Virtual system simulates the complete healthcare ecosystem, including emergency departments, specialized wards, and surgical suites.

8.4.1.3 Remote Monitoring and Diagnostics

Monitoring and diagnostics of patients through wearable devices, sensors, and IoT (Internet of Things) technology, patient health data can be continuously collected and analyzed as required (Satija et al. 2017). By implementing ML and AI algorithms, we can analyze this data in real time to detect anomalies, monitor vital signs, and predict health risks. This information will enable early investigations to explore intervention, proactive care management, and personalized treatment plans. Also, this will encourage patients to actively participate in their own healthcare while minimizing the need for frequent in-person visits.

Virtual patient care in Meta-Health revolutionizes the traditional healthcare system by utilizing modern digital technologies and virtual environments. It enhances accessibility, convenience, and patient-centricity while optimizing healthcare resources and improving outcomes.

8.4.2 Simulated Medical Training

Another vital application of mimicking healthcare within the Meta-Health framework is simulated medical training. It provides healthcare professionals with immersive and realistic learning experiences that replicate various aspects of medical practice. The following are key applications within simulated medical training:

8.4.2.1 Virtual Reality (VR) for Surgical Training

Surgeons can utilize this platform to practice and refine their skills that simulate real-world surgical scenarios (Aziz 2018; Bhugaonkar et al. 2022). This allows surgeons to perform virtual surgeries multiple times, practice intricate techniques, and gain experience in a risk-free environment, for example, the use of a VR simulator in laparoscopic surgery, where learning models were established for continuous evaluation of training processes (Lee et al. 2024). The benefit of VR is that this technology offers a safe and controlled space for skill development, team coordination, and decision-making, eventually enhancing surgical proficiency and patient safety.

8.4.2.2 Augmented Reality (AR) for Medical Education

This technology is employed to overlay virtual information in the real-world environment, enhancing medical education and training (Kamphuis et al. 2014). AR applications offer interactive and contextual information during brainstorming sessions including medical procedures, examinations, or educational sessions (Ovunc et al. 2021). For example, AR can be used to overlay anatomical structures of organs and tissues onto a physical patient, facilitating better understanding and visualization of complex medical concepts (Jin et al. 2021). Enabling interactive learning experiences, virtual demonstrations, and remote collaboration among medical professionals.

8.4.2.3 Simulation-Based Skills Development

This system utilizes advanced models and simulation techniques to replicate medical scenarios and foster skills development (Kneebone 2003). Healthcare professionals can practice their clinical skills, decision-making, and critical thinking in a controlled and realistic environment. High-fidelity patient simulators, task trainers, and virtual patient cases are used in simulation-based training to mimic clinical encounters, diagnosis processes, and treatment interventions.

For example, in one of the studies in the Netherlands, obstetric teams were trained in teamwork skills-based simulated system of crew resource management principles. After the training, patient-reported quality of care significantly improved, particularly in areas related to communication, leadership, planning, and information provision (Truijens et al. 2015). This suggests that multi-professional team training can enhance patient care quality. This platform enables repeated practice, immediate feedback, and the opportunity to learn from errors, thereby enhancing competence and confidence in various medical domains.

Simulated medical training in Meta-Health leverages cutting-edge technologies to create effective learning experiences for healthcare professionals. By mimicking real-world medical scenarios, VR, AR, and simulation-based training offer safe, accessible, and scalable methods. These methods are helpful for skill development, knowledge acquisition, and continuous education. Additionally, these technologies enhance the knowledge and expertise of healthcare professionals to improve patient health.

8.4.3 Digital Twin Technology in Healthcare

Within the Meta-Health framework, digital twin technology is a novel idea with enormous potential to change the way healthcare is delivered (Chen et al. 2023). It builds a digital twin or replica of a real-world object, like a patient, an organ, or a healthcare system. Real-time monitoring, analysis, and optimization are made possible by this technology. Key uses of digital twin technology in healthcare include the following:

8.4.3.1 Concept and Benefits of Digital Twins

In the medical field, digital twins allow for a thorough understanding of each patient (Wickramasinghe et al. 2021; Barresi et al. 2023). Through comprehending digitally stored patient-specific data, medical history, genetic data, and physiological parameters. Insights into the patient's condition, response to treatment, and overall health trajectory are obtained through the ongoing updating and analysis of this data. The advantages of digital twins—predictive analytics, personalized medicine, better clinical decision-making, and improved healthcare delivery—are all included in this technology (Pavithra et al. 2022).

8.4.3.2 Real-Time Monitoring and Predictive Analytics

Real-time monitoring of a patient's vital signs, physiological parameters, and the course of their illness is made possible by digital twins (Barresi et al. 2023). Digital twins can anticipate health outcomes, identify anomalies, and identify early indicators of decline by utilizing advanced analytics and machine learning algorithms.

8.4.3.3 Personalized Treatment Planning and Optimization

Digital twins combine predictive models, medical expertise, and patient-specific data to improve the planning, scheduling, and execution of individual treatment (Hassanien et al. 2022; Ghatti 2023). Using this method, medical practitioners can assess the efficacy of interventions and create customized treatment plans based on the unique characteristics of each patient, allowing them to simulate different treatment scenarios (Barresi et al. 2023; Menon et al. 2023). Genetics, lifestyle, comorbidities, and treatment responses are just a few of the variables that digital twin technology takes into account to help make better decisions while lowering healthcare costs and raising patient satisfaction.

Digital twin technology in Meta-Health enables healthcare providers to access information of patients, enabling personalized and proactive healthcare delivery. Real-time monitoring, predictive analytics, and personalized treatment planning optimize patient care, enhance clinical decision-making, and contribute to the overall improvement of healthcare outcomes. By utilizing these capabilities, Meta-Health can bring healthcare into a new era of precision medicine, data-driven interventions, and optimized healthcare delivery.

8.5 Future Directions and Opportunities

8.5.1 Advancements in Virtualization Technologies

The field of virtualization technologies is rapidly evolving and will further enhance the capabilities of mimicking healthcare in Meta-Health. These advancements include the following:

8.5.1.1 Enhanced Virtual Reality (VR) Experiences

Virtual reality technology is becoming more realistic advancements in VR hardware and software will enable more accurate simulations, improved haptic feedback, and realistic representations of healthcare environments. This will eventually enhance the quality of healthcare professionals and patient care.

8.5.1.2 Augmented Reality (AR) Integration

Future advancements in AR will enable healthcare professionals to visualize medical data, patient records, and diagnostic images in real time. This integration of AR with mimicking healthcare will enhance the ability of critical clinical decision-making, facilitate guided procedures, and improve the accuracy of medical interventions.

8.5.1.3 Holographic Displays and Telepresence

Holographic displays offer three-dimensional visualizations; these displays coupled with telepresence technologies enable remote collaboration and consultation among healthcare professionals from any remote location. Holographic representations of patients, medical devices, and anatomical structures will enable accurate assessments and facilitate real-time discussions, leading to improved healthcare outcomes.

8.5.2 Integration of Artificial Intelligence and Machine Learning

The integration of AI and ML will unlock new possibilities and opportunities for personalized, efficient, and precise healthcare delivery. Here are some potential areas where AI and ML will make a significant impact.

8.5.2.1 Intelligent Diagnosis and Decision Support

AI algorithms can analyze vast amounts of patient data including medical images, test reports, and health records to assist healthcare professionals in diagnosing diseases with high accuracy. Machine learning models that are trained on massive datasets can be utilized to identify patterns, spot abnormalities, and provide real-time decision assistance. By combining AI and ML, we can improve diagnosis precision, lower error rates, and provide individualized therapy suggestions.

8.5.2.2 Predictive Analytics and Early Intervention

Using medical records, family histories, lifestyle characteristics, and external variables, AI and ML systems can detect and forecast who is more prone to develop certain disorders. This preemptive strategy reduces risks and optimizes medical results, paving the way for early intervention, preventative measures, and targeted medical treatments.

8.5.2.3 Personalized Treatment and Precision Medicine

AI and ML facilitate the development of personalized therapeutic strategies by accounting for each patient's distinct traits, genetic profiles, reaction to treatment, and continuous tracking data. With the use of these technologies, complex datasets can be analyzed to determine the best course of action for each patient. This can include monitoring and adjusting dosages as well as making medication recommendations that are specific to their needs.

Redefining healthcare through the integration of cutting-edge virtualization technologies, AI, and ML has enormous potential to transform the way healthcare is provided. These developments will pave the way for more accurate, tailored, and immersive healthcare experiences, which will boost clinical decision-making, improve patient outcomes, and completely change the healthcare sector in the Meta-Health era.

8.5.3 Expansion of Digital Twin Applications

By building virtual twins of patients, healthcare systems, and procedures, digital twin technology holds the potential to completely transform the healthcare industry. It is anticipated that digital twins in healthcare will grow in a number of domains.

8.5.3.1 Disease Modeling and Predictive Analytics

Healthcare practitioners can better understand disease dynamics, stages of progression, and outcome prediction by using digital twins to simulate the progression of diseases within virtual environments. Digital twins can offer important insights into the course of a disease, the effectiveness of a treatment plan, and any potential side effects by combining patient-specific data, genetic information, and environmental factors. In order to improve patient outcomes, this information can facilitate early interventions, optimize interventions, and support individualized treatment planning.

8.5.3.2 Virtual Clinical Trials

Digital twins provide the opportunity to conduct virtual clinical trials, where new techniques, treatments, or therapies can be simulated and tested on virtual patients. Traditional clinical trials are costly and time-consuming. This strategy can lower expenses, quicken the pace of research and development, and yield more thorough information about the safety and effectiveness of treatments.

8.5.3.3 Healthcare System Optimization

Digital twins can be used to build virtual representations of clinics, hospitals, and the procedures involved in providing healthcare. By using these replicas, inefficiencies can be found, resource allocation can be optimized, and patient flow can be enhanced. Digital twins can assist healthcare organizations in making data-driven decisions to improve operational efficiency and patient experience by analyzing real-time data, such as patient volumes, staff availability, and equipment utilization.

In conclusion, digital twins present fresh possibilities for system optimization, virtual clinical trials, and illness modeling. They also facilitate the transition to virtual and remote patient care, as well as personalized and precision healthcare. Healthcare providers can improve patient care, improve operational effectiveness, and stimulate innovation in healthcare delivery models by adopting digital twin technology.

8.6 Conclusion

This chapter examines the potential for Meta-Health to transform healthcare by highlighting its role. A model of healthcare imitating virtualization, machine learning, artificial intelligence, and simulations is presented. This establishes the framework for cutting-edge medical solutions. Digital twins, simulated training, and virtual patient care are some of the applications that improve education and healthcare.

8.6.1 Summary of Mimicking Healthcare in Meta-Health

This chapter examines the idea of imitating healthcare in the context of Meta-Health, which combines the metaverse with healthcare. The definition of mimicking healthcare includes virtualizing healthcare services, simulating physical systems, and utilizing AI and simulation techniques, and the necessity of creative business models to satisfy the demands of the digital age is also highlighted. Digital twins, medical education, and virtual patient care are a few applications that allow for individualized care and remote care. Digital twins, AI, and virtualization advancements present promising opportunities. The use of mimicking in healthcare has consequences for organizations, patients, and professionals. In summary, it is a paradigm shift in healthcare that is revolutionizing virtual system optimization, training, and patient care.

8.6.2 *Key Takeaways and Implications.*

1. The integration of Meta-Health presents novel prospects and breakthroughs in healthcare.
2. Virtualization, replication, artificial intelligence, and simulation are used in Meta-Health to mimic healthcare.
3. Personalized treatment planning, training, and virtual care are the main uses.
4. Technological developments promise innovation in the provision of healthcare.
5. The consequences for organizations, patients, and professionals include data-driven decision-making and upskilling.

8.6.3 *Future Outlook and Recommendations*

1. Technology Advancements: Improve virtualization, AI, and simulation for realistic healthcare experiences.
2. Data Security and Privacy: Prioritize patient data security and privacy in digital healthcare.
3. Interoperability and Standardization: Establish standards for seamless virtual healthcare integration.
4. Ethical Considerations: Develop guidelines for ethical AI use in healthcare.
5. Regulatory Frameworks: Adapt regulations for virtual healthcare safety and ethics.
6. Collaborative Research: Promote interdisciplinary collaboration for innovative solutions.
7. Education and Training: Train healthcare professionals for virtual care competence.

These recommendations shape the future of mimicking healthcare in Meta-Health, revolutionizing healthcare in the metaverse with innovation, collaboration, and ethical practices. By considering these future outlooks and recommendations, the field of mimicking healthcare in Meta-Health can continue to advance and revolutionize. Embracing innovation, collaboration, and ethical practices will be vital in shaping a future where virtual healthcare becomes an integral part of our healthcare ecosystem, improving outcomes, accessibility, and patient experiences.

References

Al-Ghaili AM et al (2022) A review of metaverse's definitions, architecture, applications, challenges, issues, solutions, and future trends. IEEE Access 10:125835–125866

Alwasel A, Stergioulas L, Fakhimi M, Garn W (2021) Assessing patient engagement in health care: proposal for a modeling and simulation framework for behavioral analysis. JMIR Res Protoc 10:e30092

Amini R, Lisetti C, Yasavur U, Rishe N (2013) 2013 IEEE international conference on healthcare informatics. IEEE, Piscataway, pp 46–55

Aziz HA (2018) Virtual reality programs applications in healthcare. J Health Med Inform 9:305

Bansal G, Rajgopal K, Chamola V, Xiong Z, Niyato D (2022) Healthcare in metaverse: a survey on current metaverse applications in healthcare. IEEE Access 10:119914–119946

Barresi G et al (2023) Digital twins and healthcare: quick overview and human-centric perspectives. In: mHealth and human-centered design towards enhanced health, care, and well-being. Springer Nature Singapore, Singapore, pp 57–78

Bashir AK et al (2023) A survey on federated learning for the healthcare metaverse: concepts, applications, challenges, and future directions. arXiv preprint arXiv:2304.00524

Benedicta B, Caldwell PH, Scott KM (2020) How parents use, search for and appraise online health information on their child's medical condition: a pilot study. J Paediatr Child Health 56:252–258

Berros N, El Mendili F, Filaly Y, El Bouzekri El Idrissi Y (2023) Enhancing digital health services with big data analytics. Big Data Cogn Comput 7:64

Bhugaonkar K, Bhugaonkar R, Masne N (2022) The trend of metaverse and augmented & virtual reality extending to the healthcare system. Cureus 14:e29071

Chavda VP, Patel K, Patel S, Apostolopoulos V (2023) Artificial intelligence and machine learning in healthcare sector. In: Bioinformatics tools for pharmaceutical drug product development. Wiley, New York, pp 285–314

Che Z, Purushotham S, Khemani R, Liu Y (2015) Distilling knowledge from deep networks with applications to healthcare domain. arXiv preprint arXiv:1512.03542

Chen J, Yi C, Okegbile SD, Cai J (2023) Networking technologies for enabling human digital twin in personalized healthcare applications: a comprehensive survey. arXiv preprint arXiv:2301.03930

Chengoden R et al (2023) Metaverse for healthcare: a survey on potential applications, challenges and future directions. IEEE Access 11:12765–12795

De Abreu Lourenco R, Haas M, Hall J, Viney R (2017) Valuing meta-health effects for use in economic evaluations to inform reimbursement decisions: a review of the evidence. PharmacoEconomics 35:347–362

Dingler T, Kwasnicka D, Wei J, Gong E, Oldenburg B (2021) The use and promise of conversational agents in digital health. Yearb Med Inform 30:191–199

Ellahham S, Ellahham N, Simsekler MCE (2020) Application of artificial intelligence in the health care safety context: opportunities and challenges. Am J Med Qual 35:341–348

Ghatti S et al (2023) Digital twins in healthcare: a survey of current methods. Arch Clin Biomed Res 7:365–381

Gopika G, Raghuveer V, Krishna V (2022) A mini-review: everything you need to know about food deserts. J Environ Sci Public Health 6:65–68

Graafland M, Schraagen JM, Schijven MP (2012) Systematic review of serious games for medical education and surgical skills training. J Br Surg 99:1322–1330

Griffith SD et al (2019) Generating real-world tumor burden endpoints from electronic health record data: comparison of RECIST, radiology-anchored, and clinician-anchored approaches for abstracting real-world progression in non-small cell lung cancer. Adv Ther 36:2122–2136

Hassanien AE, Darwish A, Snasel V (2022) Digital twins for digital transformation: innovation in industry. Springer, Berlin

He F et al (2021) Recent progress in flexible microstructural pressure sensors toward human–machine interaction and healthcare applications. Small Methods 5:2001041

Hemingway H et al (2018) Big data from electronic health records for early and late translational cardiovascular research: challenges and potential. Eur Heart J 39:1481–1495

Jeddi Z, Bohr A (2020) Artificial intelligence in healthcare. Elsevier, Amsterdam, pp 203–234

Jin Z et al (2021) 3D printing of physical organ models: recent developments and challenges. Adv Sci 8:2101394. https://doi.org/10.1002/advs.202101394

Johansen B (2019) Data driven user experience for personalizing hearing health care. Technical University
Kamphuis C, Barsom E, Schijven M, Christoph N (2014) Augmented reality in medical education? Perspect Med Educ 3:300–311
Kasurinen J (2017) Usability issues of virtual reality learning simulator in healthcare and cybersecurity. Procedia Comput Sci 119:341–349
Kneebone R (2003) Simulation in surgical training: educational issues and practical implications. Med Educ 37:267–277
Kuo I-H, Jayawardena C, Broadbent E, MacDonald BA (2011) Multidisciplinary design approach for implementation of interactive services: communication initiation and user identification for healthcare service robots. Int J Soc Robot 3:443–456
Lee CW (2022) Application of metaverse service to healthcare industry: a strategic perspective. Int J Environ Res Public Health 19:13038
Lee S, Shetty AS, Cavuoto L (2024) Modeling of learning processes using continuous time Markov chain (CTMC) for virtual reality (VR)-based surgical training in laparoscopic surgery. IEEE Trans Learn Technol 17:462–473
Lenger AD (2022) Handbook of research on digital transformation management and tools. IGI Global, Hershey, pp 199–217
Malhotra P et al (2021) Internet of things: evolution, concerns and security challenges. Sensors 21:1809
Mans R, Reijers H, Wismeijer D, Van Genuchten M (2013) A process-oriented methodology for evaluating the impact of IT: a proposal and an application in healthcare. Inf Syst 38:1097–1115
Mendell J et al (2019) What do patients talk about? A qualitative analysis of online chat sessions with health care specialists during a "virtual" cardiac rehabilitation program. Telemed e-Health 25:71–78
Menon D, Anand B, Chowdhary CL (2023) Digital twin: exploring the intersection of virtual and physical worlds. IEEE Access 11:75152–75172
Mourtzis D (2023) The metaverse in industry 5.0: a human-centric approach towards personalized value creation. Encyclopedia 3:1105–1120
Nawawi MKM, Zulkepli J, Khalid R, Abidin N (2021) Modeling in healthcare: selection of simulation types. Univers J Public Health 9:401–409
Ngiam KY, Khor W (2019) Big data and machine learning algorithms for health-care delivery. Lancet Oncol 20:e262–e273
Ovunc SS, Yolcu MB, Emre S, Elicevik M, Celayir S (2021) Using immersive technologies to develop medical education materials. Cureus 13:e12647
Pavithra S, Pavithra D, Vanithamani R, Justin J (2022) Digital twin applications and challenges in healthcare. In: Digital twin technology: fundamentals and applications. Wiley, New York, pp 111–124
Richardson SM (2012) Toward a framework for personalized web-based training for healthcare providers in low-income countries. Stud Health Technol Inform 172:100–107
Roufaeel I et al (n.d.) Simulation modelling as a decision support tool for efficient healthcare layout design
Satija U, Ramkumar B, Manikandan MS (2017) Real-time signal quality-aware ECG telemetry system for IoT-based health care monitoring. IEEE Internet Things J 4:815–823
Senbekov M et al (2020) The recent progress and applications of digital technologies in healthcare: a review. Int J Telemed Appl 2020:8830200
Singer SJ, Benzer JK, Hamdan SU (2015) Improving health care quality and safety: the role of collective learning. J Healthc Leadersh 7:91–107
Singh K, Malhotra D (2023) Meta-health: learning-to-learn (meta-learning) as a next generation of deep learning exploring healthcare challenges and solutions for rare disorders: a systematic analysis. Arch Comput Methods Eng 30:4081–4112

Sprenger DA, Schwaninger A (2021) Technology acceptance of four digital learning technologies (classroom response system, classroom chat, e-lectures, and mobile virtual reality) after three months' usage. Int J Educ Technol High Educ 18:8
Suh I, McKinney T, Siu K-C (2023) Current perspective of metaverse application in medical education, research and patient care. Virtual Worlds 2:115–128
Thomason J (2021) Metahealth-how will the metaverse change health care? J Metaverse 1:13–16
Truijens SE et al (2015) The effect of multiprofessional simulation-based obstetric team training on patient-reported quality of care: a pilot study. Simul Healthc 10:210–216
Ullah H, Manickam S, Obaidat M, Laghari SUA, Uddin M (2023) Exploring the potential of metaverse technology in healthcare: applications, challenges, and future directions. IEEE Access 11:69686–69707
Vadlamudi S (2022) International conference on recent trends in microelectronics, automation, computing and communications systems (ICMACC). IEEE, Piscataway, pp 553–558
Veldwijk J, Johansson JV, Donkers B, de Bekker-Grob E (2017) Mimicking real life decision-making in health: allowing respondents time-to-think in a discrete choice experiment. Value Health 20:A406
Waqas M (2022) A review on meta-health–metaverse challenges and role of XAI to improve the healthcare 5.0. Int J Adv Sci Comput 1:38–42
Wickramasinghe N et al (2021) A vision for leveraging the concept of digital twins to support the provision of personalized cancer care. IEEE Internet Comput 26:17–24
Zainab HE, Bawany NZ, Imran J, Rehman W (2022) Virtual dimension—a primer to metaverse. IT Prof 24:27–33

Chapter 9
New Business Models for Meta-Health

9.1 Introduction

The integration of metaverse in healthcare has a high potential to revolutionize the industry and transform the way healthcare services are delivered. metaverse comprise virtual reality (VR), augmented reality (AR), and other immersive technologies. These technologies transform healthcare and address existing difficulties and challenges in the traditional healthcare system (Samuel 2022; Mystakidis 2022). In this chapter, we will explore the integration of the metaverse in healthcare and highlight the importance of new business models in Meta-Health.

9.1.1 Overview of the Integration of the Metaverse in Healthcare

The metaverse is the virtual world that allows users to interact with professionals in a realistic and immersive manner (Musamih et al. 2023). Rapid growth and advancements are observed in this technology which makes it immensely feasible and promising. The interactions between different groups of users open up a wide range of possibilities for improving healthcare delivery, medical training, telemedicine, data analytics, and health and wellness experiences. The main advantage of a virtual healthcare platform is to enable healthcare providers to offer services virtually, for example, consultations, remote patient monitoring, and personalized health management in a virtual environment (Chengoden et al. 2023). Another significant aspect of the metaverse in healthcare is providing virtual training and education (Tan et al. 2022). These resources can be utilized by medical practitioners by utilizing computational simulations to practice complex procedures and enhance skills, eventually improving patient health and well-being (Roufaeel n.d.). By integrating

S. Vyas et al., *Meta-Health*, https://doi.org/10.1007/978-981-96-5844-2_9

virtual medical training into existing curricula, medical schools and institutions can provide more comprehensive and effective training to future healthcare professionals.

Similarly, by providing remote consultations and healthcare monitoring, telemedicine services have also become increasingly prevalent in recent years (Chengoden et al. 2023; Field 1996; Thomason 2021). Patients can access medical care and guidance at their convenience via virtual clinics and remote patient monitoring innovations. People with physical disabilities or those who live in remote regions with no access to basic healthcare facilities will particularly benefit from this. Telemedicine services can be improved with interactive features, real-time data sharing, and improved interaction between patients and providers by using the metaverse (Bansal et al. 2022). Additionally, the metaverse offers options for data analytics, which when coupled with AI and machine learning can provide new perspectives and extensive information to enhance healthcare for patients (Bhattacharya et al. 2022; Wang et al. 2022; Ergen 2022). By improving resource allocation and promoting innovation in the sector, data-driven decision-making concerning healthcare has the potential to improve the health of patients.

9.1.2 Developing New Business Models

New business models are important as metaverse gets increasingly incorporated into the field of healthcare. Conventional healthcare business models have drawbacks when it comes to patient experience, efficiency, and availability. By incorporating the metaverse, it is possible to get over these limitations and develop cutting-edge methods for handling and delivering healthcare (Thomason 2021; Bansal et al. 2022; Anshari et al. 2023). There are multiple explanations for why Meta-Health demands new business models. Firstly, they have the potential to propel the uptake and awareness of telemedicine services, virtual healthcare systems, and other metaverse-based medications (Anshari et al. 2023). These business models could attract healthcare providers by offering these additional convenient, personalized experiences along with improved results. Second, new Meta-Health business models are able to make virtual healthcare services more economically feasible and sustainable (Periyasami and Periyasamy 2022). In order to finance the creation and maintenance of virtual platforms, medical professionals and entrepreneurs must have reliable sources of revenue. New business models can ensure the long-term sustainability and scalability of Meta-Health initiatives by developing alternative revenue-generating systems, partnerships, and collaborations (De Giovanni 2023).

New business models in the Meta-Health space may additionally promote innovation and collaboration across the healthcare system (Thomason 2021; Allam et al. 2022; Lee 2022). Multidisciplinary cooperation between technology universities, institutions, businesses, healthcare providers, legislators, and governing bodies is necessary for the incorporation of the metaverse in healthcare. This cooperative approach may lead to positive changes in the healthcare sector and accelerate the growth of Meta-Health (De Giovanni 2023; Lee 2022; Mourtzis 2023). In summary, the implementation of Meta-Health in the healthcare industry offers a revolutionary potential to transform the sector. Several choices are available in the metaverse, like unique experiences associated with health and wellness, telemedicine, data analytics, virtual healthcare networks, and virtual medical schooling. New business models need to be developed in order to take advantage of the potential of these advances in Meta-Health. These businesses have the ability to revolutionize healthcare delivery and outcomes in the digital age via fostering collaboration, ensuring financial security, and accelerating adoption.

9.2 Traditional Healthcare Business Models

Since the emergence of modern healthcare systems, traditional business models have been employed in providing care and system management. Healthcare enterprises have adopted and embraced these models (Yildirim and Sevli 2023). These models have evolved over the time to fulfil the needs of customers, medical professionals, and patients. Although they have rendered the required service, they still have intrinsic restrictions and confront the following challenges:

9.2.1 Existing Healthcare Business Models

The fee-for-service (FFS) model is one of the most recognized traditional healthcare business models (Ganapathy 2022). This approach rewarded medical professionals based on the volume and complexity of services they rendered. Since they encourage providers to offer extra services, FFS models have long been the dominant competitor. This approach might, however, lead to overuse of facilities and uneven treatment, which is a significant drawback (Letafati and Otoum 2023). Healthcare costs may increase due to the possibility of conducting unnecessary tests, operations, or treatments as professionals are paid on an individual basis. Therefore, alternate approaches such as capitation, value-based payment, and combined payments are taking the place of the FFS model (Mysore 2023). These alternative models aim to promote cost-efficiency, quality, and better health outcomes by shifting the focus from volume-based services to value-based care delivery (Maddox-Daines 2023). The traditional capitation model, which emphasizes disease management, preventive care, and cost-effective treatments within the limitations of the budget, might also be adopted as a substitute (Anderson and Rainie 2022; Morenz et al. 2023). This approach might help service providers; however, it poses difficulties for patients seeking complex or specialized care within a particular budget. In contrast, the accountable care organization (ACO) model is another one that has garnered popularity.

In this model, a collection of medical professionals collaborates to provide particular groups of patients with coordinated treatment. ACOs are typically responsible for all of the outcomes, costs, and quality of care, usually in alignment with value-based payment models. In order to improve patient outcomes, protect costs, and improve the customer experience, the model fosters integration, treatment coordination, and collaborative responsibility among providers.

9.2.2 Challenges and Limitations in the Delivery of Traditional Healthcare

It is difficult for traditional healthcare business models to adjust to the evolving demands of the industry (Farahat et al. 2023). One major problem is the fragmentation of the healthcare system, which leads to inadequacies in care communication and coordination. Furthermore, medical waste and higher costs may result from fee-for-service models' focus on volume. ACOs and bundled payment strategies are emerging as alternatives that promote value, shared accountability, and care coordination (Pandey et al. 2023). It is important that these barriers be overcome with the objective of promoting innovation and improving the provision of healthcare.

9.3 Evolution of Business Models in Meta-Health

Traditional healthcare business models find it difficult to adapt to the evolving demands of this industry. One of the primary concerns is the disintegration of the delivery of healthcare, which makes interaction and coordination of care challenging. In order to promote innovation and enhance healthcare delivery, these obstacles have to be overcome.

9.3.1 Metaverse Is Transforming Healthcare Services

The primary objective of the metaverse is to provide virtual care, such as telemedicine, digital therapies, remote monitoring, and virtual consultations (Field 1996; Bhattacharya et al. 2022; Qiu et al. 2022). These services serve as a base for technologies such as augmented reality (AR), virtual reality (VR), wearable devices (WD), and real-time data analytics (Bhugaonkar et al. 2022; Aziz 2018). With the help of these globally accessible resources, healthcare professionals can keep up-to-date records of patients and communicate with them remotely. By establishing a sense of participation and personalization that spans geographical boundaries, this metaverse virtual experience optimizes the patient experience. Additionally, the emergence of the metaverse in the healthcare sector has created a number of exciting new opportunities for entrepreneurs, tech companies, and healthcare experts (Anshari et al. 2023). For instance, these services provide a platform for interaction and collaboration between patients, healthcare professionals, and investors through virtual healthcare platforms. Millions of lives will be rescued worldwide by the chance to provide exceptional consulting and surveillance services, some of which include wellness programs, virtual clinics, digital health tracks, and support communities (Ganapathy 2022; Curtis and Brolan 2023; Miller 2023). These virtual platforms can be customized or changed to meet the demands of the patient to make it easier for them to get to the healthcare facility.

9.3.2 *The Emergence of New Business Opportunities in Meta-Health*

The metaverse has introduced innovative business models to the Meta-Health sector of the healthcare industry (Thomason 2021; Singh and Malhotra 2023). By improving their abilities and understanding in accordance with what patients and stakeholders desire, these models are assisting in transforming the way healthcare professionals work. Let us explore these developments.

9.3.2.1 Virtual Medical Training and Learning Environment

Metaverse offers a comprehensive learning environment for healthcare professionals, through virtual training that offers simulations of the surgical training modules (Graafland et al. 2012; Kneebone 2003), and real-time patient encounters, providing professionals a place to enhance their clinical abilities in a safe and immersive setting (Graafland et al. 2012; Kneebone 2003; Richardson 2012). These challenging, realistic, and interactive scenarios enable them to effective skill development. Business models for virtual medical training can involve subscription-based models, licensing fees, and partnerships with medical institutions (Sectra 2021; Kirubakaran et al. 2023).

9.3.2.2 Virtual Telemedicine Services

Integration of metaverse evolved the telemedicine services (Gajarawala and Pelkowski 2021). Remote consultations, diagnostic assessments, and continuous patient monitoring are made possible through virtual platforms. When we utilize virtual reality or augmented reality technology, we can use services particularly beneficial for individuals in remote areas or with limited mobility. Business activity utilizing monetization strategies, for example, pay-per-consultation, subscription-based models, and collaborations with healthcare insurers and employers, can be a great area to look forward.

9.3.2.3 Virtual Healthcare Marketplaces

Connecting people on the virtual healthcare marketplace platform facilitates the exchange of healthcare services, products, and information, offering appointment booking, second opinions, medical tourism, and access to specialized treatments (Bansal et al. 2022; Demir 2025). This model helps for revenue generation in healthcare marketplaces involving transaction fees, advertising partnerships, and premium service offerings.

9.3.2.4 Data Analytics and Insights

There is a huge amount of data generated within the healthcare metaverse, including patient health records and real-time physiological data, and this information can be leveraged to enable personalized medicine, predictive analytics, and population health management. This service of data analytics offers several business models that may center around offering data analytics services to healthcare organizations, developing AI-driven healthcare solutions, and collaborating with research institutions and pharmaceutical companies for data analysis and interpretation.

9.3.2.5 Virtual Health and Wellness Experiences

Immersive virtual experiences in health and wellness have emerged within the metaverse. These experiences encompass guided meditation, fitness programs, stress reduction techniques, and mental health support (Gouch 2018). Delivered through healthcare applications, they offer users an engaging environment to improve their well-being.

In conclusion, the impact of metaverse on Meta-Health is evident through its contributions to virtual medical training, telemedicine services, healthcare marketplaces, data analytics, and health and wellness experiences. As the metaverse continues to evolve, the potential for new and disruptive business models in Meta-Health will expand, shaping the future of healthcare delivery.

9.4 Key Considerations for Advanced Meta-Health Business Models

The successful development and implementation of business models in Meta-Health demands crucial factors including conducting comprehensive market analysis, identifying the precise target audience, evaluating technological requirements and infrastructure, and navigating regulatory and legal intricacies. By conscientiously addressing these aspects, businesses can strategically position themselves for the deployment of their Meta-Health business models.

9.4.1 *Market Analysis and Target Audience Identification*

Market analysis and understanding the target audience are fundamental to any successful business model (Singh and Malhotra 2023). By examining factors such as the demand for virtual healthcare services, the competitive landscape, and the distinct needs and preferences of the target audience. Analyzing user demographics, preferences, and behavior patterns enables businesses to identify specific market segments and tailor their business models accordingly. This analysis provides important insights into the profitability of the Meta-Health business model and helps to make informative decisions regarding pricing, marketing strategies, and service offerings.

9.4.2 *Technological Requirements and Infrastructure*

Meta-Health business models require an advanced level of virtual healthcare services and robust technological foundations to access the virtual platforms. High-speed Internet connectivity, secure data storage and transmission systems, and advanced software applications are essential components (Zhao 2012; Mondal et al. 2022). Selecting and integrating appropriate technologies is crucial to delivering seamless, reliable, and user-friendly virtual healthcare experiences. Businesses must evaluate their existing technological capabilities, identify the gaps, and invest in the necessary infrastructure, hardware, and software solutions to support their Meta-Health business models effectively.

9.4.3 *Regulatory and Legal Considerations*

Operating in the metaverse introduces unique regulatory challenges that may differ from traditional healthcare regulations (Lee 2022; Umar 2022; Al-Ghaili et al. 2022; Wider et al. 2023). Businesses must navigate these regulatory frameworks and be well-versed in legal implications, licensing requirements, data privacy laws, and jurisdictional considerations. This can be done by collaborating with legal experts and compliance officers; these precautions can help businesses to maintain adherence for the applicable regulations and mitigate potential legal risks (Şanlısoy and Çiloğlu 2023).

9.4.4 Ethical Considerations

Meta-Health business models require ethical consideration before designing their business plans (Chengoden et al. 2023; Bang and Kim n.d.; Chen et al. 2023). This can be achieved by safeguarding the confidentiality, security, and informed consent of patients' personal health information and securing clear guidelines and protocols for data handling (Wider et al. 2023). Transparent communication about pricing, services, and outcomes is important to foster trust among patients and stakeholders within the Meta-Health ecosystem.

In conclusion, the success of advanced Meta-Health business models relies on the strategic analysis of the healthcare market, understanding the target audience, fulfilling technological requirements, and navigating regulatory and legal complexities. Thorough market analysis enables businesses to tailor their offerings to their target audiences, coupling with technological advances to ensure the seamless delivery of virtual healthcare services. Adherence to regulatory and legal standards safeguards compliance and ethical practices.

9.5 New Business Models for Meta-Health

9.5.1 Virtual Healthcare Platforms

Virtual healthcare platforms have emerged as a crucial element of Meta-Health, capitalizing on the advancements in the metaverse (Ganapathy 2022; Waqas 2022). These platforms fundamentally transform healthcare services, providing virtual consultations, remote monitoring, and other digital healthcare solutions. The main aspects of these platforms lie in connecting healthcare providers and patients within the metaverse. In order to provide effective and tailored treatment, they offer a number of features like virtual collaboration tools, encrypted messaging, video conferencing, and access to digital medical records. Subscription-based and pay-per-service are the two typical choices accessible in terms of price and cost. Patients can access a number of services for a set charge through subscription-based models offering patients with convenience and flexibility. They may also be rewarded with special access to providers and discounted rates in exchange. Conversely, pay-per-service options serve individuals seeking particular assistance or occasional consultations while offering them more control over prices and the ability to personalize the services (Ergen 2022; Ganapathy 2022). By enhancing patient engagement and well-being and expanding their reach, these healthcare platforms also assist healthcare providers. The platforms provide access to a broader patient pool and specialized expertise by circumventing regional limitations. They also provide technologies for optimization of processes, improved interaction, and computerized booking of appointments. Selecting a virtual healthcare platform requires careful consideration of numerous factors, such as attributes, target market position, data security regulations integration capabilities with current healthcare systems, and compatibility with other platforms, all of which could contribute to improving the overall experience (Ghirmai et al. 2022).

In summary, the delivery of virtual healthcare services in the metaverse is made accessible by virtual healthcare platforms that are essential to the Meta-Health business model. They use innovative technologies to enhance accessibility, convenience, and patient experiences, ensuring regular interactions between medical personnel and patients. To make sure they choose the best platform to deliver excellent virtual healthcare services, businesses should carefully think about the cost structure, attributes, and target audience alignment.

9.5.2 Virtual Medical Training and Education

The training and education programs utilize the immersive capabilities of the metaverse to provide healthcare professionals with realistic and interactive training experiences. Professionals can utilize these training programs by leveraging advanced technologies like VR and AR. These training programs offer real-life simulations of medical scenarios, surgical simulations, medical procedure practice, diagnostic exercises, and interactive case studies, empowering professionals to refine their skills and improve patient outcomes. The benefits of these programs are manifold, such as accessibility, scalability, and the ability to replicate diverse medical scenarios effectively (Ergen 2022). In terms of business models for virtual medical training, the subscription-based model offers healthcare professionals access to a comprehensive library of virtual training modules and resources for a regular fee and expenditures. The model adopts continuous learning and professional development within the healthcare industry; alternatively, tailored training courses or certifications can be offered for a fee (Ergen 2022; Thomason 2022; Liu and Liu 2023). These programs can target specific medical specialties, advanced procedures, or emerging technologies, meeting the unique needs and interests of healthcare professionals and creating additional revenue streams.

Moreover, collaborating with medical institutions, universities, and professional organizations can enhance the credibility of virtual training programs (Ganapathy 2022; Söyler and Averbek 2022). Aligning with established institutions also provides access to wider networks and benefits from their reputation and expertise. By offering accredited courses through collaborations, businesses can attract a broader audience seeking professional certifications and continuing education credits (Yu 2022). This will help them to gain a reputation and confidence from their services, which eventually help them to establish themselves in the market and offer continuous growth and revenue generation.

9.5.3 Virtual Telemedicine Services

Virtual telemedicine services integration into the metaverse opens up new prospects for remote healthcare delivery; these services rely on digital technologies to facilitate remote consultations, diagnostics, and patient monitoring, irrespective of their physical location (Field 1996; Bhattacharya et al. 2022; Gajarawala and Pelkowski 2021; Mendell et al. 2019). This integration holds promise in overcoming geographical barriers, improving healthcare access, and enhancing patient convenience. Telemedicine can be provided in different forms, including video consultations, chat-based interactions, and remote monitoring using connected devices. These virtual platforms enable patients to securely connect with healthcare providers, seek medical advice, receive diagnoses, and undergo remote monitoring for chronic conditions. These services involve secure messaging, file sharing, and integration with electronic health records to ensure seamless communication and continuity of care.

Businesses like subscription-based models benefit patients who require regular medical check-ups or have chronic conditions that demand continuous monitoring and management. It offers them access to a network of healthcare professionals, personalized care plans, and timely interventions. Alternatively, pay-per-service models can be adopted; this model suits individuals who seek occasional medical advice or prefer a more transactional approach to healthcare. Pay-per-service options provide flexibility for patients to seek medical attention as required without committing to ongoing subscription fees. Besides, virtual telemedicine services enable remote consultations and monitoring, with subscription-based and pay-per-service models being viable options for businesses to consider. These innovative business models in Meta-Health have the potential to revolutionize healthcare delivery, enhance patient experiences, and improve access to quality care in the metaverse.

9.5.4 Virtual Healthcare Marketplaces

Virtual healthcare marketplace platforms, an emerging domain in the metaverse, act as digital ecosystems within the metaverse, facilitating the exchange of healthcare services and products (Bhattacharya et al. 2022; Ergen 2022; Bhugaonkar et al. 2022; Chen et al. 2023). Here, healthcare professionals and consumers converge to collaborate and engage in services required, and subscription fee models and transactions can be tailored as per the requirement of the customer. By bringing together healthcare providers from different specialties, patients gain access to a wide pool of experts and services (Lenger 2022). However, the revenue generation models employed by these virtual healthcare marketplaces may vary. One common approach is to charge healthcare providers a fee or commission for each transaction conducted through the platform (Jansen et al. 2018; Cruz et al. n.d.). Additionally, virtual healthcare marketplaces can also collaborate with insurance providers, pharmaceutical companies, and other healthcare stakeholders and acquire sponsorships for listings, targeted advertisements, or exclusive promotions (Tlili et al. 2023; Zhu 2022; Yao et al. 2024; Pagliai 2023).

By aligning with industry partners, these marketplaces can enhance their revenue streams while providing added value to users through special offers, discounts, or integrated insurance coverage (Chengoden et al. 2023; Veras et al. 2023). These strategic changes can help in profitable revenue generation for healthcare professions and world-class services to patients at discounted rates.

9.5.5 *Data Analytics and Insights*

Data analytics is crucial for Meta-Health business models, offering valuable insights to healthcare providers from virtual consultations, wearables, and health monitoring. For healthcare providers, Meta-Health data analytics and statistics provide deep insights into patient health trends, treatment effectiveness, and population health management (Garavand and Aslani 2022). Analyzing large-size datasets helps signature patterns, correlations, and predictive models for personalized care plans, early interventions, and preventive strategies (Shan and Shan n.d.). It also optimizes resource allocation and streamlines workflows. Recent advances in science are due to the fact that researchers can access this information and analyze patient data to identify the root cause of the diseases. The data can be obtained from clinical studies, epidemiological research, and health monitoring at scale (Yang et al. 2022), for example, bioinformatics studies on RNA and DNA sequencing can trace the early stages of cancer that can be cured or repressed on time (Kumari et al. 2023). Business models in this area may help to generate revenue, by providing data analytics services to healthcare providers. These platforms offer advanced algorithms, visualizations, and predictive models for valuable insights (Bashir et al. 2023).

Collaborations with hospitals, research institutions, pharmaceutical companies, and public health agencies also create revenue opportunities through data-sharing agreements, joint projects, or licensing arrangements. Further, this data interpretation and data analysis help to discover new medicines and cures for dangerous health problems like cancer, Alzheimer's, Parkinson's, AIDS, etc. (Pagliai 2023; Ramu et al. 2024; Bhaskar et al. 2020).

9.5.6 *Virtual Health and Wellness Experiences*

The integration of the metaverse in healthcare has generated opportunities to immersive virtual experiences focused on health and wellness. These experiences leverage VR and AR technologies to create engaging environments that promote physical and mental well-being (Yuan 2022; Liu et al. 2022). These opportunities help individuals to their health, engage in therapeutic activities, and explore self-care. They include guided meditation, stress reduction programs, fitness workouts, yoga classes, mindfulness practices, and immersive nature simulations (Ahuja et al. 2023). This environment is helpful for the individual to relax, elevate from negativity, and positively impact mental and emotional well-being. There is huge potential in generating revenues from virtual health and wellness experiences, including subscription-based access, partnerships with fitness centers, spas, health brands, and in-app purchases (Shen et al. 2021). These models provide a recurring revenue stream, while partnerships offer joint marketing and promotions opportunities, and in-app purchases allow users to enhance their experiences by buying additional content or personalized coaching. When virtual health and wellness experiences are linked with wearable devices and health-tracking technologies, it further enhances the user experience and revenue potential (Lehdonvirta 2009). Several wearable devices already utilize these resources by incorporating technology with wearable watches and health gadgets, by monitoring breathing, heart rate, and walking steps (Corchia et al. 2017). Providers can offer these services free or with premium subscriptions that include synchronized data tracking and personalized health metrics.

In conclusion, virtual health and wellness experiences in the metaverse offer engaging opportunities for individuals to prioritize their lives and well-being. Implementing revenue-based models can help to generate continuous revenue while delivering meaningful resources to the customers. These experiences have the potential to revolutionize the health industry and engage a huge number of people who need these services and are ready to pay for them, though this can be achieved by continuous efforts, creating a positive growth and learning mindset, engaging in general and customized health programs, and promoting a holistic approach to well-being in the digital realm.

9.6 Challenges and Future Outlook

9.6.1 Challenges and Future Outlook for Meta-Health Business Models

Several challenges are affecting Meta-Health's growth in implementing new business models, including:

9.6.1.1 Technological Infrastructure

Establishing and maintaining a robust technological framework for Meta-Health business models is crucial, ensuring reliable high-speed Internet connectivity, data privacy and security, and interoperability.

9.6.1.2 Regulatory and Legal Considerations

The intricate regulatory landscape necessitates compliance with privacy regulations, data protection laws, and healthcare standards, posing challenges for Meta-Health businesses. Importantly, updating regulations and creating awareness of the regulation in the industry is indeed very important for building trust and confidence for the growth of the metaverse. There are requirements of clear and transparent regulatory obligations that need to be fulfilled by the regulators and industry before initiating these businesses; otherwise, this may create havoc for the healthcare industry. The regulations should apply to consumer data security, data usage policy, and data accessibility rights.

9.6.1.3 User Adoption and Acceptance

Encouraging widespread adoption of Meta-Health business models among users is challenging, requiring efforts to build trust and educate users about the benefits and safety of virtual healthcare services. Seminars and conferences should be organized to spread awareness and confidentiality among industry and consumers to gain acceptance among the masses.

9.6.1.4 Reimbursement and Insurance Coverage

Integrating Meta-Health into the existing healthcare system raises questions about reimbursement and insurance coverage, requiring the development of suitable reimbursement models and convincing insurance providers to include virtual healthcare services.

9.6.1.5 Equity and Accessibility

Ensuring equitable access to Meta-Health services and addressing the digital divide is a significant challenge, necessitating solutions for Internet access, device affordability, and digital literacy.

9.6.2 Future Trends and Potential Advancements in Meta-Health Business Models

Several future trends can make significant improvements in the current state of business models including:

9.6.2.1 Artificial Intelligence and Machine Learning

Advancements in AI and machine learning will enhance diagnostics, personalize treatments, and improve patient outcomes through predictive analytics and decision support systems.

9.6.2.2 Virtual Reality and Augmented Reality

VR and AR technologies will revolutionize healthcare delivery, offering immersive and realistic experiences for surgical simulations and mental health therapies.

9.6.2.3 Internet of Things (IoT)

Integrating IoT devices in Meta-Health business models will enable remote patient monitoring and real-time data collection, facilitating continuous monitoring and personalized care delivery.

9.6.2.4 Blockchain Technology

Blockchain can enhance security, privacy, and interoperability in Meta-Health, enabling secure data sharing, patient-controlled health records, and transparent transactions.

9.6.2.5 Personalized Medicine

Meta-Health business models will increasingly focus on personalized medicine, leveraging data analytics and genomics to tailor treatments and interventions to individual patients.

In conclusion, while Meta-Health faces challenges in technology, regulations, user adoption, reimbursement, and accessibility, the future outlook is promising with advancements in AI, VR/AR, IoT, blockchain, and personalized medicine shaping a patient-centric healthcare system in the virtual realm.

9.7 Conclusion

9.7.1 Key Points Covered in This Chapter

In this chapter, we have discussed various aspects of Meta-Health business models and their significance in shaping the future of healthcare within the metaverse. This chapter also explores the concept of Meta-Health, which involves the integration of the metaverse into healthcare and has the potential to significantly impact the healthcare industry. By exploring innovative business models in Meta-Health, we can drive the transformation of healthcare in the digital age. The adaptation of metaverse has already begun transforming healthcare services, creating new opportunities, and revolutionizing the way healthcare is delivered. Several applications have been utilizing metaverse by providing virtual platforms for telemedicine solutions, healthcare marketplaces, and data analytics. Also, involved in enhancing the virtual health experiences of the users and creating innovative business models that are remodeling the healthcare landscape.

9.7.2 Importance of Innovative Business Models

Metaverse technologies help to revolutionize traditional healthcare delivery models by leveraging technology to enhance healthcare delivery. This new approach is improving patient health and increasing accessibility to advanced services. By doing so, they create new business opportunities for professionals and entrepreneurs, driven by advancements in technology, changing patient expectations, and the demand for personalized and convenient healthcare experiences. However, Meta-Health business models have to improve in conducting market analysis, identifying the target audience, assessing technological requirements, and addressing regulatory and legal considerations to ensure compliance with healthcare regulations. Within Meta-Health, various new business models have emerged; virtual healthcare platforms offer services through subscription-based or pay-per-service options. Virtual medical training and education programs provide opportunities for healthcare professionals to enhance their skills, with different revenue models and monetization strategies available. Virtual telemedicine services enable remote consultations and monitoring, catering to the unique needs of patients and healthcare providers.

Furthermore, data analytics offer valuable information to researchers, and healthcare providers with the support of virtual telemedicine services, patients, and healthcare professionals can get remote consultations and monitoring tailored to meet their particular demands. Furthermore, data analytics offer valuable information to researchers and healthcare professionals, and virtual marketplaces for healthcare facilitate the exchange of goods and services. With subscription-based access and opportunities for earning revenue, virtual health and wellness experiences offer comprehensive virtual experiences with a health and wellness focus. Meta-Health offers a lot of potential, but there are still challenges that need to be addressed. These challenges include legislative frameworks, technological infrastructure, security and privacy issues, and customer adoption. However, the future prospects for Meta-Health commercial models are bright. Tailored medicine, blockchain technology, augmented and virtual reality (AR), IoMT (Internet of medical things), and the integration of AI and ML are some of the potential advancements that could further revolutionize healthcare within the metaverse.

In summary, integrating the metaverse in healthcare and using advanced business approaches in Meta-Health has the potential to completely transform the healthcare industry. Healthcare in the metaverse may evolve into more patient-centered, efficient, and accessible by adopting new opportunities and overcoming the restrictions of traditional healthcare delivery. To establish the future of Meta-Health, collaboration and acceptance of these innovative business models are imperative for everyone involved in the healthcare ecosystem.

References

Ahuja AS, Polascik BW, Doddapaneni D, Byrnes ES, Sridhar J (2023) The digital metaverse: applications in artificial intelligence, medical education, and integrative health. Integr Med Res 12:100917

Al-Ghaili AM et al (2022) A review of metaverse's definitions, architecture, applications, challenges, issues, solutions, and future trends. IEEE Access 10:125835–125866

Allam Z, Sharifi A, Bibri SE, Jones DS, Krogstie J (2022) The metaverse as a virtual form of smart cities: opportunities and challenges for environmental, economic, and social sustainability in urban futures. Smart Cities 5:771–801

Anderson J, Rainie L (2022) The metaverse in 2040, vol 30. Pew Research Centre, Washington, DC

Anshari M, Syafrudin M, Alfian G (2023) Metaverse applications for new business models and disruptive innovation. IGI Global, Hershey

Aziz HA (2018) Virtual reality programs applications in healthcare. J Health Med Inform 9:305

Bang J, Kim J-Y (n.d.) International conference on human-computer interaction. Springer, Berlin, pp 367–378

Bansal G, Rajgopal K, Chamola V, Xiong Z, Niyato D (2022) Healthcare in metaverse: a survey on current metaverse applications in healthcare. IEEE Access 10:119914–119946

Bashir AK et al (2023) Federated learning for the healthcare metaverse: concepts, applications, challenges, and future directions. IEEE Internet Things J 10:21873

Bhaskar S et al (2020) Telemedicine across the globe-position paper from the COVID-19 pandemic health system resilience PROGRAM (REPROGRAM) international consortium (Part 1). Front Public Health 8:556720

Bhattacharya P et al (2022) International conference on computer, information and telecommunication systems (CITS). IEEE, Piscataway, pp 1–5

Bhugaonkar K, Bhugaonkar R, Masne N (2022) The trend of metaverse and augmented & virtual reality extending to the healthcare system. Cureus 14:e29071

Chen Z, Gan W, Sun J, Wu J, Yu PS (2023) Open metaverse: issues, evolution, and future. arXiv preprint arXiv:2304.13931

Chengoden R et al (2023) Metaverse for healthcare: a survey on potential applications, challenges and future directions. IEEE Access 11:12765

Corchia L, Monti G, De Benedetto E, Tarricone L (2017) Wearable antennas for remote health care monitoring systems. Int J Antennas Propag 2017:1–11
Cruz M, Oliveira A, Pinheiro A (n.d.) Informatics, 47
Curtis C, Brolan CE (2023) Health care in the metaverse. Med J Aust 218:46
De Giovanni P (2023) Sustainability of the metaverse: a transition to industry 5.0. Sustainability 15:6079
Demir Ç (2025) The effect of metaverse technology on medical tourism process. J Gastronomy Hosp Travel 8(1):96–102
Ergen I (2022) Design in metaverse: artificial intelligence, game design, style-Gan2 and more…. Allied Publishers, Chennai
Farahat MA, Darwish A, Hassanien AE (2023) The implication of metaverse in the traditional medical environment and healthcare sector: applications and challenges. In: The future of metaverse in the virtual era and physical world. Springer, Berlin, pp 105–133
Field MJ (1996) Telemedicine: a guide to assessing telecommunications for health care. National Academies Press (US), Washington, DC
Gajarawala SN, Pelkowski JN (2021) Telehealth benefits and barriers. J Nurse Pract 17:218–221. https://doi.org/10.1016/j.nurpra.2020.09.013
Ganapathy K (2022) Metaverse and healthcare: a clinician's perspective. Apollo Med 19:256–261
Garavand A, Aslani N (2022) Metaverse phenomenon and its impact on health: a scoping review. Inform Med Unlocked 32:101029
Ghirmai S, Mebrahtom D, Aloqaily M, Guizani M, Debbah M (2022) 2022 IEEE smartworld, ubiquitous intelligence & computing, scalable computing & communications, digital twin, privacy computing, metaverse, autonomous & trusted vehicles (SmartWorld/UIC/ScalCom/DigitalTwin/PriComp/Meta). IEEE, Piscataway, pp 2468–2475
Gouch AD (2018) Stress, coping strategies and cardiovascular disease in African American women with ethical considerations for health care practitioners. Temple University, Philadelphia
Graafland M, Schraagen JM, Schijven MP (2012) Systematic review of serious games for medical education and surgical skills training. J Br Surg 99:1322–1330
Jansen L, van Schijndel M, van Waarde J, van Busschbach J (2018) Health-economic outcomes in hospital patients with medical-psychiatric comorbidity: a systematic review and meta-analysis. PLoS One 13:e0194029
Kirubakaran SJ, Gunasekaran A, Dolly DRJ, Jagannath DJ, Peter JD (2023) A feasible approach to smart remote health monitoring: subscription-based model. Front Public Health 11:1150455. https://doi.org/10.3389/fpubh.2023.1150455
Kneebone R (2003) Simulation in surgical training: educational issues and practical implications. Med Educ 37:267–277
Kumari J, Das K, Goldust M (2023) Metaverse in diagnosis of skin diseases. J Cosmet Dermatol 5:169
Lee CW (2022) Application of metaverse service to healthcare industry: a strategic perspective. Int J Environ Res Public Health 19:13038
Lehdonvirta V (2009) Virtual item sales as a revenue model: identifying attributes that drive purchase decisions. Electron Commer Res 9:97–113. https://doi.org/10.1007/s10660-009-9028-2
Lenger AD (2022) Handbook of research on digital transformation management and tools. IGI Global, Hershey, pp 199–217
Letafati M, Otoum S (2023) On the privacy and security for e-health services in the metaverse: an overview. Ad Hoc Netw 150:103262
Liu X, Liu Y (2023) Distributed learning for metaverse over wireless networks. IEEE Commun Mag 61:40
Liu Z, Ren L, Xiao C, Zhang K, Demian P (2022) Virtual reality aided therapy towards health 4.0: a two-decade bibliometric analysis. Int J Environ Res Public Health 19:1525
Maddox-Daines K (2023) Managing people in the hybrid workplace. Taylor & Francis, Milton Park

Mendell J et al (2019) What do patients talk about? A qualitative analysis of online chat sessions with health care specialists during a "virtual" cardiac rehabilitation program. Telemed e-Health 25:71–78
Miller TW (2023) Digital health transformed for elderly care through the metaverse. IJCMCR 27(5):4
Mondal S, Singh S, Gupta H (2022) A meta-analysis of green and sustainable business models: a comprehensive approach. J Clean Prod 371:133623
Morenz AM, Zhou L, Wong ES, Liao JM (2023) Association between capitated payments and preventive care among U.S. Adults. AJPM Focus 2:100116. https://doi.org/10.1016/j.focus.2023.100116
Mourtzis D (2023) The metaverse in industry 5.0: a human-centric approach towards personalized value creation. Encyclopedia 3:1105–1120
Musamih A et al (2023) Metaverse in healthcare: applications, challenges, and future directions. IEEE Consum Electron Mag 12(4):33–46
Mysore I (2023) Digital identity in the new era of personalized medicine. IGI Global, Hershey, pp 1–27
Mystakidis S (2022) Metaverse. Encyclopedia 2:486–497
Pagliai A (2023) Personalized medicine meets artificial intelligence: beyond "hype", towards the metaverse. Springer, Berlin, pp 233–247
Pandey A, Chirputkar A, Ashok P (2023) 2023 international conference on innovative data communication technologies and application (ICIDCA). IEEE, Piscataway, pp 334–337
Periyasami S, Periyasamy AP (2022) Metaverse as future promising platform business model: case study on fashion value chain. Businesses 2:527–545
Qiu CS, Majeed A, Khan S, Watson M (2022) Transforming health through the metaverse. J R Soc Med 115:484–486
Ramu SP et al (2024) The metaverse for cognitive health: a paradigm shift. IEEE Consum Electron Mag 13(3):73–79
Richardson SM (2012) Toward a framework for personalized web-based training for healthcare providers in low-income countries. Stud Health Technol Inform 172:100–107
Roufaeel I et al (n.d.) Simulation modelling as a decision support tool for efficient healthcare layout design
Samuel S (2022) Augmented intelligence in healthcare: a pragmatic and integrated analysis. Springer, Berlin, pp 433–451
Şanlısoy S, Çiloğlu T (2023) A view of the future of the metaverse economy on the basis of the global financial system: new opportunities and risks. J Corpor Govern Insurance Risk Manag 10:28–41
Sectra (2021) Moving from a license to subscription-based model for health IT. Sectra, Linköping
Shan R, Shan T(n.d.) International conference on big data. Springer, Berlin, pp 48–63
Shen B, Tan W, Guo J, Zhao L, Qin P (2021) How to promote user purchase in metaverse? A systematic literature review on consumer behavior research and virtual commerce application design. Appl Sci 11:11087
Singh K, Malhotra D (2023) Meta-health: learning-to-learn (meta-learning) as a next generation of deep learning exploring healthcare challenges and solutions for rare disorders: a systematic analysis. Arch Comput Methods Eng 30:4081–4112
Söyler S, Averbek GS (2022) SAĞLIK TEKNOLOJİLERİ VE METAVERSE: POTANSİYEL UYGULAMA ALANLARI VE MEVCUT ENGELLER. Int Anatolia Acad Online J Health Sci 8:138–166
Tan TF et al (2022) Metaverse and virtual health care in ophthalmology: opportunities and challenges. Asia-Pac J Ophthalmol 11:237–246
Thomason J (2021) Metahealth-how will the metaverse change health care? J Metaverse 1:13–16
Thomason J (2022) Metaverse, token economies, and non-communicable diseases. Global Health J 6:164–167

Tlili A, Huang R, Kinshuk X (2023) Metaverse for climbing the ladder toward 'industry 5.0'and 'society 5.0'? Serv Ind J 43:260–287
Umar A (2022) 2022 international conference on cloud computing, big data and internet of things (3CBIT). IEEE, Piscataway, pp 160–165
Veras M et al (2023) A framework for equitable virtual rehabilitation in the metaverse era: challenges and opportunities. Front Rehabil Sci 4:1241020
Wang G et al (2022) Development of metaverse for intelligent healthcare. Nat Mach Intell 4:922–929
Waqas M (2022) A review on meta-health–metaverse challenges and role of XAI to improve the healthcare 5.0. Int J Adv Sci Comput 1:38–42
Wider W et al (2023) Metaverse chronicles: a bibliometric analysis of its evolving landscape. Int J Hum Comput Interact 40(17):4873–4886
Yang Y, Siau K, Xie W, Sun Y (2022) Smart health: intelligent healthcare systems in the metaverse, artificial intelligence, and data science era. J Organ End User Comput 34:1–14
Yao X et al (2024) Enhancing wisdom manufacturing as industrial metaverse for industry and society 5.0. J Intell Manuf 35:235–255
Yildirim E, Sevli O (2023) Importance, impact, and future potential of extended reality applications in the metaverse
Yu J-E (2022) Exploration of educational possibilities by four metaverse types in physical education. Technologies 10:104
Yuan W (2022) Identifying the effect of digital healthcare products in metaverse on mental health: studying the interaction of cyberchondria and technophobia. Am J Health Behav 46:729–739
Zhao J (2012) 2012 International joint conference on service sciences. IEEE, Piscataway, pp 281–284
Zhu H (2022) Metaaid: a flexible framework for developing metaverse applications via ai technology and human editing. arXiv preprint arXiv:2204.01614

Chapter 10
Future of Meta-Health

10.1 Introduction

As metaverse is revolutionizing healthcare and emerging as Meta-Health, many challenges setting the agenda today include the emergence of chronic diseases, aging populations, limited workforce, constraints in resources, and growing costs. In that scenario, the potentials that a metaverse can bring to healthcare are expected to be remarkable. Five key domains—medical care, wellness, collaborative practices, healthcare education, and monetization—are foreseen for the application of the metaverse. The pandemic has propelled the healthcare system toward digital revolution and normalized telehealth. With imperative social distancing and touchless interactions, telemedicine has become indispensable, necessitating the adoption of technologies like digital twinning and blockchain within healthcare. These technological facades promise original walks for augmenting treatments, improving patient outcomes, and reducing expenses (Li et al. 2024).

The digital health realm has metamorphosed to be at the fore in the realignment of care; so, it is playing a massive role in pharmaceuticals and biotechnology. Some of the predictable applications of metaverse in medicine include training modules to enhance communication skills between healthcare experts and students, promising extensive advancements in holistic healthcare encircling disease prevention and treatment (George and Kizhakkethottam 2024). The Meta-Health can continue elevating patient experiences and practitioners' effectiveness by further embracing such concepts as virtual clinics, AI utilization, augmented reality, human digital twins, medical simulations, and robotics. It is going to revolutionize medicine and healthcare (Jeong and Lee 2025). The changes that Meta-Health is going to make in patients' experiences, care provision, and general outcomes are immense. On the way to the integration of the metaverse into healthcare, not everything is smooth. Inevitably, barriers pertaining to patient privacy, data security issues, cost implications, and technical interoperability must be overcome. As this transformation unfolds, the full

S. Vyas et al., *Meta-Health*, https://doi.org/10.1007/978-981-96-5844-2_10

potential of what the Meta-Health has to offer in healthcare industry cannot happen without careful collaboration between healthcare practitioners, technologists, and policymakers (Adil et al. 2025).

10.2 Predictable Trails for Metaverse Integration in Healthcare (Making of Meta-Health)

The amalgamation of the metaverse into healthcare (Meta-Health) means potential for transformative changes (Chengoden et al. 2023). Herein, it has several future directions regarding potential applications:

- Virtual Clinics and Consultations: Leveraging AR and VR to create immersive environments that allow consultations to take place remotely. The technology would make it much easier for doctors to engage their patients more personally and intriguingly, which would improve communication and the understanding of medical conditions visually.
- Medical Education and Training: Metaverse can lend a new dimension to medical education and training. Simulation and surgical procedures in virtual environments, surrounded by realistic environments, will be the entangling for medical students and professionals alike. This will help them in decision-making and developing skills without the consequence of the real world.
- Patient Education: The metaverse would be used to design interactive and immersive experiences for improving patient education. It would enable patients to view and simulate their conditions better and the options for treatment or surgery (Ullah et al. 2023).
- Therapeutic Applications: Virtual reality experiences can be used in pain management and other mental health treatments. It is possible to divert the patient's attention from pain and anxiety in such VR environments, which helps during the process of recovery.
- Physical Rehabilitation: The metaverse could be the huge opportunity in physical therapy and rehabilitation. Patients who are recovering from injuries or surgeries can interact with their personalized exercises and activities in the VR environment, which is basically more engaging and motivating for the process of rehabilitation.
- Support Groups and Mental Health: The ability to create virtual support groups for sharing experiences and therapy sessions may establish a safe environment whereby people can communicate with others facing similar health issues. This can be paramount to those suffering from rare conditions or who cannot easily attend in-person support groups.
- Remote Monitoring and Diagnostics: The integration of wearable devices and sensors with the metaverse could provide real-time health data. Therefore, it would allow doctors to monitor remotely the vital signs and other health metrics of patients for easy diagnosis and management of conditions.

- Clinical Trials and Drug Development: Virtual simulations could make huge differences in the design of drugs and medical treatment processes. Researchers working on digital models that simulate the possible effects of the therapies could fasten the drug development process.
- Health Data Visualization: The metaverse can be used to create new ways for visualizing complex health data through depictions of the outcomes of both medical imaging and genetic information. This is an innovation that can assist doctors in making logical decisions and taking better care of their patients' health.
- Health and Wellness Gamification: The metaverse can also drive healthier routines through gamified experiences. If activities targeted toward wellness are transformed into effectively fun games, then subjects might be more motivated to take regular exercise, eat healthy food, and follow other beneficial practices.

10.3 Challenges on the Way to Metaverse Integration in Healthcare (Meta-Health)

The integration of the metaverse into healthcare, i.e., Meta-Health, presents a series of challenges that need careful consideration (Chengoden et al. 2023):

- **Patient Protection and Privacy Guidelines**: A substantial challenge lies in aligning the metaverse with patient safety and privacy regulations, such as those outlined in the HIPAA guidelines. Industry stakeholders must ensure the confidentiality of patients' sensitive information, including PHI (personal health information) and ePHI (electronic personal health information), within the metaverse context. As telemedicine and mobile device integration become more prevalent, policymakers will need to revisit and adapt HIPAA regulations to address the vast volume of data present in the metaverse (Ullah et al. 2023).
- **Elevated Setup Costs**: Realizing the full potential of the metaverse in healthcare requires substantial infrastructure investment. Finally, implementation hardware devices of advanced technology, such as eyewear, sensors, and wearables, plus uninterruptable 5G connectivity to match, may be very difficult for many physicians and healthcare facilities to afford. If the metaverse is to become accessible, the cost factor in integration must be watered down.
- **Cybersecurity Concerns**: The escalation in cyberattacks is one of the major causes of concern about protection of the patient data in metaverse. As healthcare institutions are often targeted by cyber-criminals, who find them very easy and lucrative targets, the conjunction of the metaverse with healthcare opens a whole new dimension of security threats. Besides, the increased quantity of patient data necessitates an enhanced focus on privacy. On a larger scale, the comfort level that patients feel in interacting within the metaverse remains to be seen, while initial signs appear promising.

- **Interoperability Challenges**: Realizing interoperability in a non-steady-state environment is quite challenging. The addition of a new aspect of the metaverse may bring new implications for devices that have been developing their interoperability with other devices through different platforms and by different networks. For this reason, the metaverse would probably be gradually implemented and may require new standards for data communications that are specific to the special needs of the medical field.

10.4 Ongoing Meta-Health or Metaverse Healthcare Projects

- **Osso VR**: Osso VR provides a surgeon with immersive surgical training simulations in VR. It allows surgeons to practice medical procedures, improving patient outcomes with hands-on experience in building the required skills.
- **Cedars-Sinai Medical Center—VR Pain Management**: Cedars-Sinai Medical Center treats the pain of patients during medical procedures with the use of VR. The more the immersive VR experience, the less the pain and anxiety, therefore reducing the dosage and usage of traditional pain medication.
- **Virti**: Virti combines virtual reality, artificial intelligence, and data analytics to provide healthcare professionals with training and education. The platform offers realistic medical scenario simulations to enhance decision-making skills.
- **KindVR**: KindVR focuses on addressing patients' psychological and emotional needs through virtual reality. The platform offers relaxation experiences and calming environments to reduce stress and anxiety.
- **Surgical Theatre**: Surgical Theater provides surgeons with 3D virtual reality reconstructions of patients' anatomy using medical imaging data. This aids surgical planning and patient understanding of procedures.
- **Psious**: Psious offers virtual reality exposure therapy for mental health conditions. Controlled virtual environments aid patients in confronting and managing phobias, anxiety, and posttraumatic stress disorder.
- **Oxford Medical Simulation**: Oxford Medical Simulation provides virtual reality scenarios for medical training. Medical professionals can practice clinical scenarios in immersive VR environments, enhancing diagnostic and decision-making skills.
- **Mursion**: While not exclusive to healthcare, Mursion's virtual reality platform focuses on soft skills training, including communication and empathy. This has potential applications in healthcare settings requiring effective patient interaction.
- **Brain Power**: Brain Power employs augmented reality glasses to assist individuals with autism in improving social and communication skills. The project has potential therapeutic applications.

These examples demonstrate the diverse applications of the metaverse, using virtual and augmented reality technologies to address training, patient engagement, mental health, and more within the healthcare sector (Zoccarato et al. 2024).

10.5 Meta-Health in the Next 10 Years

Predicting the exact advances in the healthcare over the next 10 years is challenging, but we can predict some potential developments based on current trends and emerging technologies (Uppamma et al. 2025). Here is a hypothetical outlook on how the metaverse might be integrated into healthcare within the next decade:

- **Advanced Virtual Clinics**: Virtual reality (VR) and augmented reality (AR) are prepared to become inherent to medical discussions. By submersing specialists in practical virtual environments, these technologies will augment diagnoses and enhance communication with patients.
- **Global Access to Medical Expertise**: The metaverse could help in bridging geographical gaps in healthcare. Patients can easily reach out to specialists and medical experts across the world, especially for rare diseases and specialized treatments.
- **Personalized Treatment Plans**: AI, in collaboration with data analytics, will personalize treatment plans for the metaverse using data from wearable devices, genetic profiles, and medical histories to individualize health outcomes.
- **Immersive Medical Training**: Medical education will shift to immersive metaverse simulations, in which medical students and professionals will do mock surgeries, diagnose diseases, and manage emergencies in very realistic virtual environments.
- **Real-Time Health Monitoring**: Seamless combination with wearable devices and sensors into the metaverse will facilitate continuous health monitoring, whereby patients' real-time vital signs and health metrics would create quicker responses to changes in health.
- **Therapeutic VR/AR**: VR will play a significant role in pain management, rehabilitation, and mental health treatments. The immersive experience will create a nice way of distracting patients from the pain, aiding in physical therapy, and delivering therapeutic interferences against mental health challenges.
- **Precision Medicine Advancements**: The metaverse will drive breakthroughs in precision medicine. AI-driven simulations will enable the prediction of how individual patients will respond to various treatments so that the doctor can select the most appropriate therapeutic approaches.
- **Collaborative Medical Research**: The metaverse, with its virtual environments, would provide a collaborative space for researchers across disciplines and locations. This collaboration will speed up the discovery of new treatments, medical technologies, and therapies.
- **Ethical and Regulatory Considerations**: As the metaverse is implemented in healthcare, robust regulations and ethical frameworks will be necessary. Protecting the privacy of the patients, guaranteeing data security, responsible utilization of technologies will become most paramount.
- **Telemedicine and Telehealth Service Evolution**: The development of telemedicine will go beyond the simple video calling to include immersive virtual visits. In this scheme, patients will be able to virtually "visit" clinics, hospitals, or even

pharmacies, therefore transforming the concept of remote healthcare experiences. The metaverse is going to further the area of telehealth services to the extent of even conducting remote surgeries by robotic systems controlled by surgeons sitting at other locations.
- **Healthcare Gamification**: Gamified health experiences within the metaverse will drive healthier behaviors through virtual challenges, incentives, and social collaborations that promote regular exercise, balanced nutrition, and treatment adherence.
- **Medical Data Management**: Decentralized technologies like blockchain will secure medical records, conceding patients control over their health data. It will involve secure sharing with healthcare providers.

Although these opportunities are interesting, it will take technological advancement and regulatory support, ethical reflections, and industrial collaboration to attain them. Integration of metaverse in healthcare will not happen overnight but will follow an evolution path over the next decade.

10.6 Prerequisites of Meta-Health (Metaverse New Business Models) for All Stakeholders

Every healthcare company will have to create a new business model that includes the metaverse for remaining sustainable. A few items to ponder, related to just how large of a disruptor the metaverse will be to health care, includes the following:

- Insurers may choose to pay/reimburse for virtual health visits differently than an in-person visit.
- Misconduct litigations may involve recording the time spent in the metaverse for accountability resolutions.
- Commercial payers will require to develop unique medical codes for the metaverse-focused sessions.
- Software vendors will require their devices and software to be compatible with the metaverse for healthcare.
- There needs to be a real discussion regarding whether physicians can specify medication and/or treatment virtually.

10.7 Beyond Meta-Health and More…

The integration of the metaverse in healthcare, i.e., Meta-Health, is likely to have a profound and transformative impact on the industry (Musamih et al. 2022). Beyond the initial adoption and implementation of metaverse technologies, several potential developments could shape the future of healthcare:

- **Hyper-personalized Healthcare**: The metaverse's analysis of extensive patient data will drive personalized healthcare. Treatment plans, interventions, and preventive measures will be tailored based on individual genetics, lifestyle, and health data (Rane et al. 2023).
- **Predictive and Preventive Medicine**: The metaverse can democratize access to healthcare using AI and data analytics, enable early disease recognition, and allow for interventions. Individual data-based predictive models detecting health risks could result in proactive measures against illness.
- **Remote and Home-Based Healthcare**: The metaverse will augment remote monitoring and diagnostics, hence helping to deliver quality care to patients within their homes. Wearable devices and sensors will track key health metrics uninterruptedly for interventions at appropriate times.
- **Global Medical Collaboration Networks**: This could eventually lead to virtual and augmented realities being used for real-time collaboration between medical professionals from across the globe in complex case consultation, sharing of insights, or even assistance in surgeries that transcended geographical borders (Uppamma et al. 2025).
- **Virtual Health Records and Interoperability**: The metaverse can bring ease to health records by making them very user-friendly and accessible. Patients would be capable of managing their records securely while ensuring interoperability among healthcare systems, improving care coordination.
- **Decentralized Healthcare**: Blockchain and decentralized technologies offer an infrastructure that provides patients with self-sovereignty over health information, thereby providing secure and transparent sharing and rebuilding trust in relationships between patients and their healthcare providers (Bansal et al. 2022).
- **Continual Learning and Upskilling**: Healthcare experts can indulge in continuous education and training on the metaverse. It would provide access to the most recent advancements in medicine, shared experience, and collaboration with peers across worldwide.
- **Healthcare Gamification and Behavioral Change**: The probability of receiving virtual rewards, challenges, and social interaction because it gamifies healthy behaviors will drive prolonged participation to induce people to make positive changes in life.
- **Bioethical Considerations**: As the metaverse finds a place in healthcare, concerns regarding data privacy and consent will arise, and questions regarding AI's part in making medical decisions call for deep reflection.
- **Health Ecosystem Integration**: The metaverse might impeccably integrate patients, providers, pharmaceutical firms, insurers, and researchers to foster collaboration and innovation in health ecosystems.
- **Regulatory Evolution**: The metaverse converging into healthcare will give rise to new laws and standards that will provide patient safety, health data security, and ethical consumption.
- **New Business Models**: The metaverse would be able to incubate new models and opportunities in healthcare. It can indeed disrupt traditional models of healthcare delivery, freeing up space for innovative startups and collaborations.

These are some of the potential developments that are indicative of the transformative power of Meta-Health promising innovation through varied domains of patient care, research, education, and regulation (Díaz-Chieng et al. 2022).

10.8 Upcoming Projects for Implementing Metaverse in Healthcare

This section includes a list of some significant upcoming projects determined on executing the Meta-Health (Adil et al. 2025). These projects are still under progress, exhibiting the expanding interest and investment in this area:

- **Nvidia's Clara Platform for Medical AI in the metaverse**: Nvidia is going to extend the Clara platform with more advanced AI-driven tools for medical imaging, virtual consultations, and surgical simulations in the metaverse. In this respect, the platform will be designed to offer real-time data processing and visualizations for healthcare experts.

  Impact: More accurate diagnoses and increased efficiency, better training environments for surgeons and radiologists, and more immersive telemedicine experiences.
- **Virtual Reality Medical Centers by HTC VIVE**: HTC has collaborated with several healthcare providers in the construction of VR-based centers in medicine. This will include psychological counseling, rehabilitation, and even virtual consultations.

  Impact: Healthcare services accessibility is expected to increase to a high level for those staying in remote areas and more engaging treatments against mental health.
- **Immersive Therapy Solutions by AppliedVR**: AppliedVR is extending its VR-based solutions for therapeutic purposes into the metaverse, targeting the management of chronic pain and mental health. Its platform will have the ability to engage patients with personalized treatment plans in virtual environments.

  Impact: Nonpharmacological pain management options, increased patient engagement in therapy, and improved mental health outcomes.
- **Metaverse Health Hub by Meta (formerly Facebook)**: Meta is reportedly exploring the creation of a "Metaverse Health Hub," whereby patients will be able to communicate with healthcare providers, gain access to medical information, and participate in wellness programs in a virtual environment.

  Impact: Better engagement of patients in healthcare, wellness programs tailored to individual patient needs, and a new model for preventive care.
- **Decentralized Healthcare Ecosystem by Aimedis**: German blockchain-based healthcare platform Aimedis is currently developing a decentralized healthcare ecosystem within the metaverse. The whole concept of this project is to network patients, healthcare providers, and researchers in a safe virtual space.

  Impact: Higher level of patient autonomy, better security of data, and increased collaboration worldwide in medical research and treatment.

- **Virtual Medical Training Platforms by SimX**: SimX is a growing VR medical simulation platform to includes more comprehensive training modules for the different medical specialties. These modules shall be plugged into the metaverse to allow for much more collaborative and immersive training experiences.
  Impact: Improved medical education and training, reduced errors in clinical practice, and more confident, competent healthcare professionals.
- **Remote Rehabilitation Programs by XRHealth**: XRHealth is currently developing metaverse-based rehabilitation programs that can enable patients to carry out exercises for their treatment in various virtual environments. This would be tailor-made and scalable for many kinds of rehabilitation needs.
  Impact: Increased accessibility to rehabilitation services, increased adherence of patients to therapy, and more effective rehabilitation outcomes.
- **Holomedicine Association's Virtual Hospital**: Holomedicine Association will create a metaverse-based virtual hospital concept, in which healthcare professionals could train for complex surgery, collaborate for research, and even virtually have congresses to debate new techniques in medicine.
  Impact: Improvement of collaboration among health professionals, improvement in surgical outcomes, and faster medical innovation.
- **Augmented Reality Diagnostics by Magic Leap**: Magic Leap integrates augmented reality with the metaverse to come up with next-generation diagnostic solutions. Advanced tools of this sort will allow health professionals to view patient data and diagnostics in 3D for accurate diagnosis.
  Impact: Much more accurate and faster diagnostics, improved patient outcomes, and a new standard in how medical data would be visualized.
- **Global Virtual Health Community by Roblox**: Roblox is developing a global virtual health community inside its metaverse platform. It would bring users into an environment that is gamified, including health education, wellness programs, and support groups of peers.
  Impact: It will increase public awareness and education regarding health issues, improve access to wellness resources, and build stronger patient communities.

10.9 Conclusion

Meta-Health in collaboration with its immersive technologies like VR and AR holds substantial potential for converting diverse characteristics of the healthcare industry. It spans from personalized treatment plans to immersive medical training, real-time health monitoring, therapeutic interventions, and even global medical alliance. Challenges need to be addressed include patient privacy concerns, cybersecurity issues, and interoperability hurdles. The next decade could observe advanced virtual clinics, with breakthroughs in precision medicine and an expansion in telehealth services, driven by AI, data analytics, and the underlying regulatory framework. More significantly, the effect of the metaverse on health is no longer going to be marked by the technological uptake alone but has started influencing predictive medicine, decentralized healthcare, and ethical deliberations in reforming how patients, specialists, and stakeholders involve in the context of healthcare.

References

Adil M, Song H, Khan MK, Mastorakis S, Farouk A, Jin Z (2025) Metaverse in health care: security challenges and pathways for future research. IEEE Syst Man Cybernet Mag 11(1):95–106

Bansal G, Rajgopal K, Chamola V, Xiong Z, Niyato D (2022) Healthcare in metaverse: a survey on current metaverse applications in healthcare. IEEE Access 10:119914–119946

Chengoden R, Victor N, Huynh-The T, Yenduri G, Jhaveri RH, Alazab M et al (2023) Metaverse for healthcare: a survey on potential applications, challenges and future directions. IEEE Access 11:12765–12795

Díaz-Chieng LY, Auza-Santiváñez JC, Castillo JIR (2022) The future of health in the metaverse. Metaverse Basic Appl Res 1:1

George L, Kizhakkethottam JJ (2024) Unleashing the future of healthcare in the metaverse: the pivotal role of blockchain in data privacy. In: Examining the metaverse in healthcare: opportunities, challenges, and future directions. IGI Global, Hershey, pp 77–102

Jeong E, Lee D (2025) Metaverse applications in healthcare: opportunities and challenges. Serv Bus 19(1):4

Li Y, Gunasekeran DV, RaviChandran N, Tan TF, Ong JCL, Thirunavukarasu AJ et al (2024) The next generation of healthcare ecosystem in the metaverse. Biom J 47(3):100679

Musamih A, Yaqoob I, Salah K, Jayaraman R, Al-Hammadi Y, Omar M, Ellahham S (2022) Metaverse in healthcare: applications, challenges, and future directions. IEEE Consum Electron Mag 12(4):33–46

Rane N, Choudhary S, Rane J (2023) Healthcare metaverse: applications, challenges, and future development

Ullah H, Manickam S, Obaidat M, Laghari SUA, Uddin M (2023) Exploring the potential of metaverse technology in healthcare: applications, challenges, and future directions. IEEE Access 11:69686–69707

Uppamma P, Padma A, Chithanuru V, Ravula V (2025) Metaverse in healthcare: applications and challenges. In: Exploring the metaverse. Elsevier, Amsterdam, pp 45–68

Zoccarato F, Ghezzi A, Lettieri E, Toletti G (2024) Technological scanning for foresight: the case of metaverse applications for healthcare. Futures 164:103476

GPSR Compliance

The European Union's (EU) General Product Safety Regulation (GPSR) is a set of rules that requires consumer products to be safe and our obligations to ensure this.

If you have any concerns about our products, you can contact us on ProductSafety@springernature.com

In case Publisher is established outside the EU, the EU authorized representative is:

Springer Nature Customer Service Center GmbH
Europaplatz 3
69115 Heidelberg, Germany

Batch number: 10726135

Printed by Printforce, the Netherlands